Endangered Species

Carolina Academic Press
Ethnographic Studies in Medical Anthropology Series

Pamela J. Stewart
and
Andrew Strathern
Series Editors

Endangered Species

Health, Illness and Death Among
Madagascar's People of the Forest

Janice Harper

CAROLINA ACADEMIC PRESS
Durham, North Carolina

ISBN: 0-89089-238-5
LCCN: 2002107086

Carolina Academic Press
700 Kent Street
Durham, North Carolina 27701
Telephone (919) 489-7486
Fax (919) 493-5668
www.cap-press.com

Printed in the United States of America

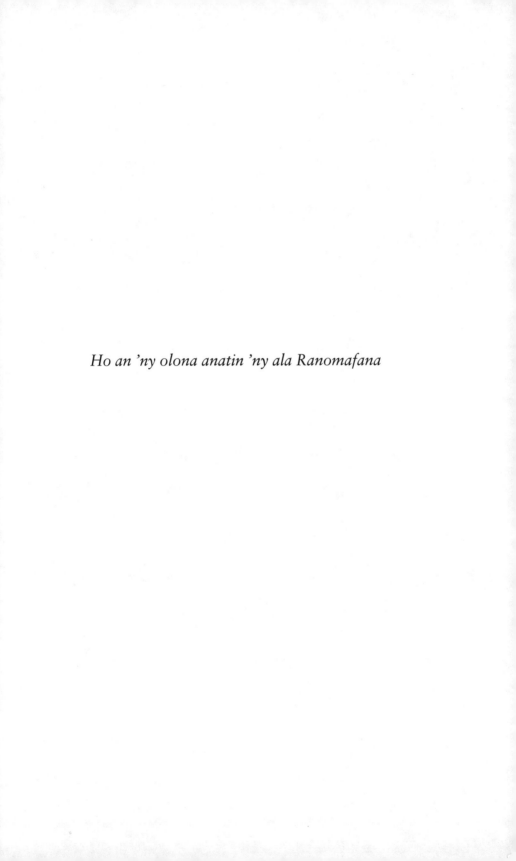

Ho an 'ny olona anatin 'ny ala Ranomafana

Contents

Series Editors' Preface

Medical Anthropology Series:
Endangered Species
Health, Illness and Death Among
Madagascar's People of the Forest

Pamela J. Stewart and
Andrew Strathern

Harper's book presents a fascinating narrative of the Malagasy living in Ranotsara who live in the southeast of Madagascar. This presentation provides the reader with a vivid picture of how these people cope with contemporary changes in their world. The materials are contextualized in terms of the historical background of the research area, emphasizing the environmental concerns of the people and their interaction with the local National Park Project.

These Malagasy forest farmers, like many peoples around the globe, have an intimate and sustained relationship with their physical environment in addition to deep-seated emotional perceptions of their landscape. The focus here on the environment and how this overlays with health issues is particularly insightful in terms of both physical and psychological wellness.

Harper's arguments throughout the book also reflect the increasing concern that anthropologists have to understand better the dynamics of the wider contexts in which the lives of people are set. Her work resonates well with studies conducted in other places. For example, the Duna people of Papua New Guinea, with whom we work, live their lives with a tangible awareness of the intertwining aspects of their environment and their society at large (see Stewart and Strathern 2002).

The discussion of Harper's interactions with the Ranaomafana National Park Project is a valuable part of this work. It highlights the growing awareness by anthropologists that fieldwork experiences nowadays are often impacted by the presence of governmental, company or non-governmental agencies that are involved in development projects locally within the field area (see Stewart and Strathern 2001). Often one aspect of the interaction of development projects within an area is the provision of health care services of one sort or anther. Harper's discussion of the problems that arose among the Malagasy living in Ranotsara from these services (or lack thereof) is a cautionary tale which unfolds through the chapters of her book.

We are very pleased to present Janice Harper's book as the latest contribution to the Ethnographic Studies in Medical Anthropology Series. The other titles in this Series include:

> "*Curing and Healing: Medical Anthropology in Global Perspective*", 1999 (by Andrew Strathern and Pamela J. Stewart)

> "*Healing the Modern in a Central Javanese City*", 2001 (by Steve Ferzacca)

> "*Physicians at Work, Patients in Pain*, 2nd edition", 2001 (by Kaja Finkler)

References

Stewart, Pamela J. and Andrew Strathern (eds.) 2001. *Anthropology and Consultancy*. Special Issue of *Social Analysis* (University of Adelaide, Australia).

Stewart, Pamela J. and Andrew Strathern 2002. *Remaking the World: Myth, Mining, and Ritual Change among the Duna of Papua New Guinea*. Washington, D.C.: Smithsonian Institution Press.

November 2001
Department of Anthropology
University of Pittsburgh
Pittsburgh, PA 15260 USA

Acknowledgments

Rather than wait until the end of a long list of people to thank for having contributed to this book, I would like to offer my profound gratitude right up front to the people of the village I call Ranotsara, for having invited me into their homes and hearts. One of the most difficult issues I have grappled with in writing this book has been how to present intimate details of people's lives in a way that will reveal important social, economic and political tensions regarding the use of land, resources, and medicines, but to do so in a manner consistent with the warmth and respect I have felt for the residents of Ranotsara. Unfortunately, I know that I will have failed in many respects, and that there are statements and representations that I have made that would disturb some people. For any distress or injustice this writing causes, I am profoundly sorry. For any misunderstandings or inaccuracies I have presented, I am equally sorry and hope that I or others will have the opportunity to correct such distortions. I do trust, however, that this presentation of the village and its residents is a true and accurate account of my observations and interpretations of the research problem. I hope, too, that my presentation reflects the complexity and vitality of the people of Ranotsara who, for the rest of the world, will remain anonymous.

While all among those with whom I lived were very kind, some stand out for having provided particular support and friendship. Pierety cooked my meals, washed my dishes, hauled my water, pounded my coffee and managed the details of living in a rainforest that were incomprehensibly time-consuming in my eyes. She freed me for the mundane work of interviews, and in the process, she became a major conduit into the lives of the farmers with whom I lived. She patiently explained the world in which I had entered, translated complex Tanala speech into something I could comprehend, humored me, and put up with me. Marie-Jacqueline and Seraphine likewise provided great comradery and assistance. Seraphine, in particular, kept me laughing with her keen sense of humor and theatrics. Benoit, who I have sadly learned has since passed away, and I were continually bickering over such things as firewood and cow heads, but he was a friendly and likeable nemesis just the same who will forever remain in my heart. Mira is a comedic delight and a woman of great grace; I am proud to have named my daughter in her honor. Botovao and Raymond provided much support and helpful insights into their world. Tonga, Vesa, and Lehavana patiently complied with my elementary interrogations into their professions as *ombiasa*. iFakandro, Vaohita, Toandro, Botokely and Kotolehibe were fine *mpanjaka* who carried their roles with dignity and grace; the deaths of Botokely and Kotolehibe were great losses to the world in which they allowed me to enter. Kalapiso, Willy, Philomene, Jean-Chris, and Reoly were brilliant and charming children who were a real joy to work with and learn from. And Manga was so charming and funny that I miss him every day.

Many of my social science colleagues who have worked, and continue to work, in Madagascar, have provided me with personal and professional support in a number of ways. In some cases, though we have barely met, if at all, they have shared their data and insights in order that the social issues of Madagascar become as important to researchers as the biological research. In other cases, they have shared not only their data and insights, but many rich conversations and social support. These many colleagues whose work has enriched my own and, I hope, the lives of the Malagasy, include Sarah Fee, Paul Ferraro, Lisa Gezon, Paul Hanson, Sabrina Hardenbergh,, Edgar Krebs, Pier Larson, Narivelo Rajaonarimanana, Lesley Sharp, Linda Sussman, and Wendy Walker.

Special thanks go to Joe and Dai Peters and Dan and Elizabeth Turk, for sharing their homes, research, and friendship amidst the turbulence of Ranomafana, and in the years since then.

Professor Pierre Verin, of the *Institut National des Langues et Civilisations Orientales* in Paris, France, deserves more gratitude than I can express in these few lines. He has not only devoted his life and profession to expanding the ethnographic knowledge of Madagascar, he has provided ongoing and invaluable assistance to scholars of Madagascar. By opening his home and library to me and to so many others, Professor Verin and his family have given to scholarship and humanity a great gift. I also thank the staff and faculty of the *Institut National des Langues et Civilisations Orientales* for their patience, support and assistance during my residence in Paris and association with their school.

In Antananarivo, as I initiated my study of the Malagasy language and conducted archival research, I received considerable hospitality and assistance from more generous people than I can ever recall. Among them were Jean-Aime Rakatoarisoa of the *Musee d'Art et Archaeologie*, the family Ramanakasina, Rakoto Ratsimamanga, Etienne Rakotobe and Corneille Rasolomananana of the *Centre National de Recherches Appliques Pharmacutique*, and the enigmatic and engaging Peter Robinson, to whom I owe a special gratitude.

I will always have profound appreciation and respect for Dr. Bezaka Jules Bosco and Lorena Bezaka of the Ranomafana National Park Project. Lorena's great warmth, humor, and research assistance helped a great deal, both professionally and personally. And Dr. Bosco's dedication to healing and caring for his patients is an honor to his profession.

Several people helped me with translations, research, and interviews. Among them, I thank Chantelle, who I foolishly drove away with my madness, Razafimandimby Voangy, whose good cheer and sage advice helped temper me, Soandro whose English, wit and versatility were a Godsend, and Rodin, whose chosen path should take him far. I also received helpful advice, translations, and historical information from Flaurent, of the Ranomafana National Park Project Museum, and from George. I apologize for not having had the grace to take down your last names. Madame Lillia Rakotaelson and Jeannette Razananirina Mohammed helped me to learn Malagasy and were both dedicated and inspiring teachers. Monique Rodriguez of Cortez Travel helped me to get around the world with minimal fuss and often with little notice, and the staff at the Station Thermal became a family to me as I awaited my research clearance.

I would not have been able to carry out this research had it not been for the generous support of private and public donors. Language and academic studies were funded by U.S. Department of Education Title VI Foreign Language and Area Studies (FLAS) fellowships, awarded through the Michigan State University Center for Advanced Studies in International Development (CASID). Predissertation training and research was supported by the Social Science Research Council International Predissertation Fellowship Program, with funding provided by the Ford Foundation and the American Council of Learned Societies. The dissertation fieldwork was supported by a Fulbright Institute for International Education Year-Abroad Fellowship, a National Science Foundation Dissertation Improvement Award, the Michigan State University College of Social Science, M.S.U. International Studies and Programs, and the M.S.U. Women and International Development Program. Dissertation write-up was supported by the M.S.U. College of Social Science. The University of Houston provided me funding for research assistance during the write up of this book, as well as a job which enabled me to devote the time necessary to complete it.

My parents, Clifton and Neela Harper, provided me more than I ever expected, both personally and financially, in their support of this research project. I will be forever sorry that they could not live to see their generosity rewarded by the completion of this book. I also thank my brother Alan "Zoky" Harper, and sister, Elizabeth Harper, for not throwing me out of the house while I began writing this book, and I thank Michael Skladany for providing financial support during the early stages of this writing.

Eva Spinner provided considerable insight and assistance, undertaking some of the most tedious portions of this book, including preparing the index. Diane Shea generously volunteered to prepare the genealogical chart from my nearly incoherent notes.

Members of my dissertation committee provided considerable advice throughout the research and writing process, as well as provided a number of suggestions on how to organize and write this book. These mentors include Drs. Anne Ferguson, Laurie Medina, Rita Gallin and Barbara Rylko Bauer. My theoretical orientations and methodologies were particularly enriched by the guidance of my dissertation advisor, Dr. William Derman. Although he does not appear in this book, he visited the village on two occasions and offered substantial advice and direction; my gratitude to his continual support and counsel cannot be overstated.

My editors, Dr. Pamela Stewart and Dr. Andrew Strathern of the University of Pittsburgh, and Dr. Leah Rutchick of Carolina Academic Press, provided exceptional guidance in cleaning up the manuscript, strengthening my arguments, and helping to make this book both readable and scholarly. I would like to especially thank these editors, and the publishers at Carolina Academic Press, for publishing this story in its entirety, without ever having asked me to expurgate passages that could potentially risk political critique, encouraging me, instead, to use it as an opportunity for demonstrating to students of anthropology the complexities of practicing anthropology in the context of development. And the readers of this book owe much of its clarity to the fine eye of Dr. Sheryl Mc-Curdy whose copy-editing helped weed out much of the tedium and redundancy with which I had originally infested it. Thank you, Sheryl.

Professors Maurice Bloch and Pier Larson read earlier drafts of this work; their suggestions and critiques were right on target and helped to strengthen the work, any weaknesses in this final product are mine alone.

There are multitudes of others, too numerous to include here, who have assisted me and supported me. To those whose contributions I have failed to include, I apologize.

While so many have contributed in small and large ways into the making of this book, the errors, weaknesses, judgements, and interpretations are mine alone.

And finally, I need to acknowledge that a real price was paid by this research, and it was paid by the Malagasy people. One hundred and eighty village residents and a staff of Malagasy project employees were caught in the middle of an expatriate battle for control — control over information and ideas. I wanted information to test my ideas, and the Project administrators wanted to control what information I accessed, and what ideas I expressed. In this struggle for control, we each put our own respective interests for personal success ahead of the needs of the Malagasy farmers who hosted our stay on their lands. Most perversely, we did so under the illusion that we were helping them.

It is not another "research project" that the people of Madagascar need. I hope, however, that for all the shortcomings of this research project, it will mark the first step toward my own efforts to repay my hosts for their kindness, generosity, and the lessons that I learned from them.

Endangered Species

Chapter 1

Introduction

What follows is a story about how people living amidst some of the last remnants of the lush and captivating forests of the world struggle to survive amidst greater struggles beyond them, struggles which engage them in strange and unexpected ways. It is about people who are neither apart from nature nor one with it. It is about people who use plants, barks, and roots from the forest to treat diseases that are mostly curable, but not necessarily by plants, barks, and roots. Yet their continual reliance on the forest's botany for their health care is less conditioned by their "culture" than it is by social inequalities that have rendered them cash poor and resource rich. The resources that surround them, however, are controlled by others, others who seek not to harm, but to help, and in so "helping" they have intensified the unequal divisions of land and labor that have enabled some to rise, and others to fall.

In telling the story, I show first, how conservation of the forests of Madagascar have contributed to unequal access to land, labor, and cash income, and therefore, to greater illnesses for many, who must often rely on plant medicines when more effective treatments are unaffordable. Second, I contend that the relationship between health and environment is neither uniformly experienced by residents, nor mediated by "tribal" or "ethnic" beliefs. Instead, I argue that the ways that people experience and view their health in terms of their environment are shaped more significantly by other social identities, including age, gender, and lineage. Third, the ways that people live in the forest and use its resources are not the stuff of "tradition," but instead, must be understood within their historical and social contexts.

I have entitled this book, "Endangered Species" not to suggest that the Malagasy are faced with extinction; indeed, their cultural integrity persists despite two centuries of European, and now American, social engineering. The title is intended to draw attention to the fact that biodiversity *includes* humans, and to the proclivity of thinking of the rainforest in terms of non-humans who are endangered. The dangers which confront the Malagasy who live in the forest may not be the threat of extinction, but do include the threat of high mortality, debilitating disease, malnutrition and chronic poverty. While a group, be it an "ethnic" group or a lineage, is unlikely to die out, a family may well face the threat of losing all its members to early, and avoidable, deaths.

Thus, this ethnography challenges many common views about the rainforest, about its conservation, and about the people who inhabit it. But as an ethnography, the social actors I present include not only those who live in the forest, but those who craft and carry out the environmental and social policies that affect the forest residents. In this way, the story is not only about the people of Madagascar, but about the people of the United States and other people in positions of power, as well. To understand the views and practices of the Malagasy, one must also reflect on the views and practices of those who seek protection of the forests, toward what ends, and at whose expense.

Backdrop

From April 1995 to June 1996, I lived in a small village in the southeastern region of Madagascar, among people self-identified as "Tanala," or people of the forest.[1] When I first arrived, approximately 180 people lived in the thirty homes that comprised Ranotsara, a community that found itself at the nexus of local, national, and international concerns when a national park—funded and administered by international donors—was established at its doorstep. Surrounding the village are irrigated rice fields reaching to the fringes of old growth rain and cloud forest, as well as large tracts of previously forested land that have been cleared for swidden agriculture. Historical processes of colonialism, migration, and economic change have contributed to the changing ecology over the village's one hundred year history.

When, in 1990, what remained of the forest was enclosed as the Ranomafana National Park, Ranotsara was selected as one of the twenty-six pilot villages of the Ranomafana National Park Project (RNPP). The RNPP was established through a grant agreement between Duke University and the United States Agency for International Development (USAID). Although celebrated as a national park of Madagascar, the land and its resources were managed by the World Bank-funded *Association National des Gestations et Areas Protegee* (ANGAP) [National Association for the Management of Protected Areas], which controls all national parks and protected areas in Madagascar. The park was further subject to the policies of the USAID-funded Ranomafana National Park Project which em-

---

1. Many of the villagers are descended from ancestors of the Betsileo ethnic group, and claim kinship ties to Betsileo residents of other communities outside the forest. As such, while all agreed that Ranotsara was ethnically identified as a Tanala village, and its residents practiced the Tanala way of life, many also identified themselves as simultaneously Tanala and Betsileo. These issues regarding ethnicity and descent are discussed in Chapters Four and Five.

ployed American administrators to design and direct the social, economic, agricultural, and scientific strategies aimed at protecting the biodiversity and species habitat of the region. While Malagasy citizens were employed at many levels of administration, the vast majority came from urban areas outside the region of Ranomafana, while project design, decision making, and resource allocation primarily remained the privilege of Americans.

Despite this foreign control, the objectives of the project and the intentions of foreign administrators were in no way intended to harm the Malagasy people. Indeed, the national park and project came about from a genuine concern to better the world, both socially and ecologically. Nonetheless, as I show in this book, the theoretical assumptions concerning the relationships between environment and culture, which guided the Ranomafana National Park Project and continue to guide national parks throughout the world, undermined the very social and ecological objectives of its creators, and had profound implications for the African people of the region.

The strategies of the project aimed at protecting the environment included encouraging significant changes in the economic and agricultural practices of local residents of the 26 selected pilot villages. In exchange for "economic development," residents of these villages were to relinquish what they considered to be their ancestral forest lands for use as a national park. Believing that the region's biodiversity was threatened by encroaching "slash and burn" rice farming (more accurately termed "swidden," and indigenously termed "*tavy*") pilot villages in the project were offered technological assistance to shift from swidden to irrigated agriculture. It was believed by project administrators that *tavy* was an unsustainable agricultural strategy that would have to be abandoned if the forest were to survive. As such, administrators reasoned that if encouraged to adopt other forms of agriculture, provided with alternative economic strategies such as eco-tourism, and educated about the rarity and importance of their native biology, residents would either cooperate in abandoning *tavy*, or have no legitimate justification for continuing the practice.

With the creation of the Ranomafana National Park Project, the Ranomafana area became, not for the first time, host to foreigners and urban-based elite Malagasy who have historically been viewed by those living in rural areas more as foreign oppressors, than as national compatriots. The arrival of the foreigners has, however, also brought with it the opportunity for some people to prosper from commerce with the outsiders. In the town of Ranomafana, which is centrally located in the forested area, those who own restaurants, hotels, or Western-styled housing have been advantaged, while prices for local goods and produce have increased beyond the purchasing ability of most local residents. Hanson (1997:41,42) notes that over the last five years, prices in the Ranomafana market have skyrocketed. People in Ambodiaviavy believe that these increases are due to the numerous *vazaha* (foreigners) attending the market. Ecological tourists from all over the world visit the RNP and before entering the forest, stock-up with provisions bought at the local market. Believing that most *vazaha* "have wealth" (*manan-karena*), the salespeople raise the prices of fruits and vegetables. These merchants are then reluctant to sell such produce to area residents as they are never sure when the next tourist will arrive.

Hanson further points out that of these merchants working in the Ranomafana market, only two claimed that their ancestral lands were located in the region; the remaining were merchants from large cities and primarily identified with the Merina ethnic group of the central highlands.

While the project promoted an image of empowering local communities through economic development, beneficiaries were not necessarily those who have relinquished rights to the forest. The project made no secret of its "trickle-down" approach, in which prosperity of local elites is considered a first-step toward economic development.

> Many programs are top-down or bottom-up, but the middle should also not be ignored. Skilled entrepreneurs and businessmen can be helpful in implementation. If these people feel the project is assisting the local economy, they can give useful advice and assistance (Wright 1993:18).

Recognizing that local residents do not generally respect the authority of outsiders, the project hired local residents to "monitor" the agricultural practices and forest activities of their families and neighbors. With fines and, in a few cases, imprisonment, having limited success, the project incorporated a coercive element into its plans.

> Attempts to protect some of the remaining forests by creating a national park, however, brought us directly up against the villagers. For the people of Madagascar, our preservation efforts were obstacles to their use of their own natural resources. They use forest products such as thatch for the construction of houses, as food, and as medicines, and of course they clear the forests for crop land.
>
> Therefore we went around to each of the small villages in the area and explained to the villagers that we wanted to help them preserve their wildlife *and would be willing to make an exchange for their cooperation with the Department of Water and Forestry* (Wright 1990:452, emphasis added).

Thus, when the National Park was established, use of the forest was prohibited. As such, further shifting cultivation of forested land was and remains prohibited, along with collecting fuel wood, fish, medicinal plants, hunting, or foraging. But while residents are prohibited from entering the forest within the Park boundaries, they do not necessarily stay out. Instead, foraging and swidden rice cultivation have continued, though illicitly. Only researchers, scientists, and people purchasing a permit are legally permitted to enter the forest. At the time of my fieldwork, the cost of a permit to enter the forest was approximately $15—clearly beyond the purchasing ability of a local resident who might make as little as 30 cents a day. What to a forest farmer was his or her ancestral land, to be used when needed or to be passed to one's children, is now land that outsiders decree he or she can no longer even walk upon, no matter how many decades one has lived in the shade of the forest's trees. But a tourist or a researcher like myself can arrive from Antananarivo or "Andafy," a mythical land where all the (mostly) white people come from, and spend a day in the forest enjoying its pristine beauty, or a year there earning a living or a degree.

Organization and Objectives of the Ranomafana National Park Project

The aim of the Ranomafana National Park Project (RNPP) was

to preserve the biological diversity and ecosystems of the park through a program linking conservation of the core park area with improved standards of living and income alternatives within the surrounding peripheral zone (RNPP 1994:2).[2]

---

2. The "peripheral zone" has proven to be an elastic concept in the minds of park administration. Initially, it was to include any village or community within five kilometers of the Park boundaries. During my stay, Park administrators told me that the peripheral zone would be reduced to three kilometers, because this was shown to be the zone which most impacted the forests in the region, while at the same time, I was informed by one senior project administrator that the peripheral zone of the park had been *extended* to include all regions in the southeast to ensure that any research undertaken complied with the objectives of the project (Director of RNPP Antananarivo Office, personal communication, January 1995). When residents of Ranotsara sought project assistance for health and agricultural projects, they were sometimes told that they no longer resided in the peripheral zone, and therefore, were ineligible for such assistance, while surveillance of their farming activities continued. Residents were not at all clear on whether or not they were "within" the peripheral zone, nor was I, despite my numerous questions in this regard. Indeed, it was my impression that the peripheral zone was at any time from three

The project was intended to provide administrative and technical support during the early stages of the park, in order to ensure its long-term success.[3]

> The objective of this project is to help preserve the biological diversity and ecosystems of the newly created Ranomafana National Park through an integrated program linking conservation of the core park area with sustained development within a surrounding buffer zone. The project seeks to: (1) prevent further degradation of natural resources through alternatives to slash and burn agriculture, (2) increase agricultural and forest productivity, (3) strengthen Malagasy institutions and technical and research capacity, and (4) study and analyze the area's rich biology (USAID n/d:8).

The project was organized into two phases. Phase I (1990-1993) was a planning and design phase, in which comprehensive baseline socioeconomic and biological data were to have been collected, the park boundaries established and demarcated, the infrastructure developed, and the peripheral zone development activities implemented. It was at this stage that twenty-six villages were targeted as "pilot villages" to participate in conservation and development activities and receive strategic and financial assistance. Phase II (1994-1996) was intended to "build on the research, data collected, and lessons learned during the first phase of the project... successful on-going activities will be continued in the original pilot villages while some project activities may extend beyond the 5km peripheral zone to provide a regional perspective and approach" (RNPP 1994:i).

> A central tenet held in the creation of the park is that it does not exist in a vacuum. People living in the peripheral zone are integral parts of the ecosystem, and it is recognized that biological diversity of the core area can be preserved only if local residents benefit from and actively participate in the management of area resources. In order to progress towards the project goal of **conservation of biological diversity and ecosystems of Ranomafana National Park**, the objective of the RNPP during Phase II is:

---

to twenty-five kilometers from the Park boundaries, depending upon the objectives of the project.

3. From 1990 to 1995, the *Association Nationale pour la Gestion d'Aires Protégées* (ANGAP), funded by USAID and the World Bank, though maintaining its identity as a national institution was responsible for implementing the national plan for biodiversity protection and training, and for coordinating the peripheral zone development activities. From 1995 to the present, it has taken the lead in managing the park itself, as well as overseeing the continued operations of the project.

> To diminish human pressures on the protected area through the introduction of sustainable agricultural systems, alternative income sources, and the sound management of natural resources of local communities.
> Means to the objective include the implementation of an integrated conservation and development project linking sustainable management and utilization of natural resources with increased socio-economic levels of residents in the peripheral zone (RNPP 1994:ii, emphasis in the original).

Project activities included increasing the productivity of staple and market crops, facilitating sustainable utilization of forest products, initiating alternative means of income generation, developing non-consumptive alternatives to forest use (particularly eco-tourism), and developing a protected area infrastructure.

> The central theme in the RNPP will be the linkage of forest and natural resources to improved socio-economic conditions. By establishing this linkage through project activities, it is anticipated that local residents will have an increased awareness of the value of natural resources, that local residents will perceive empowerment over the management of area resources, that they will gain incentives for conservation of the resource and the project goal can be achieved (RNPP 1994:ii).

The Project sought to transform the economic structure of the region from one based on subsistence hillside farming to one based on commodity production, with a heavy emphasis on wet-rice paddy production, eco-tourism, and international marketing of renewable resources. In so doing, it adopted the rhetoric of participatory, sustainable development. How villagers were to be integrated into the Project remained problematic, but integration was initially sought through the (loosely-defined) participation of the twenty-six original "pilot villages," one of which was Ranotsara.

> ...we went around to each of the small villages in the area and explained to the villagers that we wanted to help them preserve their wildlife and would be willing to make an exchange for their cooperation with the Department of Water and Forestry. Their responses revealed just how low their levels of public health actually were. Above all, they wanted access to medicines and to hospitals; they had no medical facilities at all, but they wanted their people to be healthy (Wright 1990:452,453).

The villagers of Ranotsara remember well the 1986 visit of the Principal Investigator of the Project. "She came here with a notebook and she was very friendly," Faly, a village leader recalled, "She told us we could no longer go into the forest or burn *tavy*. She said if we stayed out of the forest, they would help us. She asked us what we needed, and we told her there was much sickness, we needed doctors and medicines. And we told her our school needed supplies, and if we did not burn *tavy*, we needed chemical inputs and fertilizers for the *tanim-bary* [irrigated rice agriculture], and jobs for people who do not have *tanim-bary*. She wrote everything down, and then she drank some *toaka* [homemade rum] with us, and she left. We never saw her again, but after that, some doctors came to see how sick we were."

Faly's wife, Nirina, picked up the conversation at this point. She was very excited and, as often with her, laughing so hard she could hardly keep from coughing and hacking. "Yes, the doctors came, and they all had plates with them. They were very nice plates, like the white ones you have," she said, laughing, hacking, and pointing a shaking finger in my direction, as she referred to my white enamel covered tin plates.

"We thought they were very nice *vazaha* [foreigners], to give everyone these plates," she continued between fits of strong, deep coughing, "we thought at first they were like the missionaries, to give us such a nice gift. And every family got enough plates for each of their children. But then they told us what they wanted us to do with them!!!" Nirina and all present began to laugh hysterically at the memory of a team of public health specialists who distributed plates to be used to collect fecal samples from children in order to measure parasitical loads.

> We began by conducting a survey of the villagers in order to determine exactly what their health needs were; the results painted a grim picture indeed. Water in the villages contains all manner of waterborne diseases. Fifty percent of the people had malaria during the cold season when you couldn't even find a mosquito. Infant mortality is extremely high, and half of the children are malnourished; 97 percent of the children had worms of some sort. Sanitation levels are practically nonexistent (Wright 1990:453).

> So we are implementing alternative agricultural practices that allow rice paddies and forests to coexist; we are educating the villagers about basic sanitation and health care; we are encouraging ecotourism as a source of additional income and, therefore, as a preservation incentive; and we are exchanging ideas with the villages and integrating their techniques, knowledge and perspectives into our problem-solving approaches (Wright 1990:453).

The creation of the Ranomafana National Park, like the creation of national parks throughout the world, arose not only from the legitimate scientific concern for species preservation in the face of human consumption of the ecological habitat, but also from a cultural aesthetic in which "nature" is separated from "culture." The idea that the environment is something separate from the people that inhabit it is a distinctly Western concept, and is not a view shared by all societies. Recent Western thought has separated people from the environment in such a way that humans are perceived as either controllers of the environment, or destroyers of it. At the same time, the environment is viewed as something beyond the control of humans, something that controls and destroys seemingly passive humans (Croll and Parkin 1992). These approaches analytically divide people from their environments, and tend to privilege one, while subordinating the other.

Thus divided, tropical forests have come to be regarded as "pristine," the product of natural change, rather than human action. Indeed, as the melodies of lemurs, birds, and laughter united the forest with the homestead, the human with the wild, I was calmed and quieted. And the lush, multi-shaded greens of the foliage against the ruddy-reds of the earth, the blinding blue of the sky, and the deep, dark umbers of the faces of my friends, all mingling with the fragrance of flowers, rainfall, and roasting coffee, struck me as a heavenly beauty unparalleled in the States.

Yet the "pristine beauty" of the tropical forest obscures the discomfort and distress that come of living and working in the tropical environment. Pain, disfigurement, illness and death are endured by all whose lives are marked by relentless work and intensifying poverty, in the humid and rain-soaked environment in which some forms of life which thrive are neither rare nor beautiful. Bacteria, viruses, parasites, rats, and deadly mosquitoes flourish alongside the exotic—and indeed endangered—lemurs, frogs, butterflies and birds that have so captured the hearts of those who live outside the tropics.

Recognizing the severity of health problems and the widespread concern that "development" include health care for residents of the region, the project promoted itself as a potential source of such care. Thus, in addition to agricultural assistance, villagers were also to receive access to Western medical care by way of a traveling health team which would periodically visit each village, and they were promised economic assistance to repair schools and expand the educational opportunities in the region.

Health care was initially provided to residents of Ranotsara, via monthly visits by a physician and nurse who dispensed pharmaceutical medicines and treated chronic and acute illnesses. In this way, access to Western medicines was directly linked to relinquishing access to the forest; indeed, residents were discouraged from using indigenous medicines, as the health team at that time disparaged plant and other indigenous medicines as "backward" (D. Peters 1994a). But by 1993, after three years of the monthly visits, the health care abruptly stopped, with no explanation or warning to the villagers. Project administrators explained to me that health care was terminated because local conflicts made it too problematic to carry out the project's agricultural objectives in this village (Project Manager, personal communication 1995). The former physician for the health team, who had been responsible for making the monthly visits, explained that he did not receive any support for health care activities and when his contract expired, his work was terminated (Project Physician, First Phase, personal communication 1996). The American Conservation Director informed me that in his opinion the only relationship between health and conservation was that in order to conserve the forest, population growth needed to be controlled. Thus, because most of the women refused to use the birth control pills offered by the health team, he reasoned that the project had no obligation to continue health services (Conservation Director, personal communication, 1996). Nonetheless, the project did continue to support the idea of exploring the possible commodification of plant medicines as a means toward sustainable development of the region's ecosystem (RNPP 1994).

At the same time that visiting health care in this village ceased, other significant regional changes took place. In 1990, Madagascar entered into the first phase of the National Environmental Action Plan (NEAP), which linked economic development to conservation. The first component of this program was a land privatization campaign directed by the World Bank, which reached the Ranomafana region a few years later. Some villagers appropriated land that had been farmed by their neighbors by having it registered to themselves, while others complained that their taxes increased when they registered their land. Structural adjustment programs imposed by the International Monetary Fund to relieve the country's debt, included the devaluation of the Malagasy Franc to half its previous value. The Gulf War caused petrol prices to escalate, and a cyclone caused considerable damage to village homes and obstructed access to urban markets. Rapid inflation drastically changed the local economy; some community members, who for historical reasons had more land than others, benefitted by this inflation, while the majority suffered.

Prior to the mid- to late-1980s, such economic distress would have been mediated by clearing more forest land. Instead, by the early 1990s, such distress was exacerbated as further clearing was prohibited. Moreover, those already advantageously positioned by their greater economic power benefitted by the project's assistance in the shift to irrigated rice agriculture because they had access to suitable lands, while the rapid inflation provided them with the low-cost labor of their economically impoverished neighbors. They were further advantaged because they had the capital to invest in fertilizers and chemical inputs. Consequently, within a period of a few years, the social structure of the village changed from one in which all households had access to forest land and labor for subsistence agriculture, to one in which the majority of the households worked as agricultural wage laborers for a minority controlling irrigated rice fields producing a surplus for sale at market.

During this period of rapid social change, and right on the heels of the abrupt departure of the traveling physician, illnesses and deaths escalated considerably, while access to pharmaceutical medicines was sharply curtailed. Most people no longer had the purchasing power to buy pharmaceutical medicines, which had been introduced through health programs of the French colonial state. While I had expected that those who could no longer purchase pharmaceutical medicines would rely more on plant medicines, this did not necessarily occur. With the introduction of pharmaceutical medicines and ideas about health and disease as grounded in biology, which were promoted in the nineteenth and first half of the twentieth centuries by the colonial government and by Lutheran and Catholic missionaries, the role of the *ombiasa* (diviner/healer) appears to have shifted from diviner and healer, to primarily diviner, treating more cosmological illnesses than "illnesses of God" or "illnesses of age."[4] I believe that this changing role of the *ombiasa* as one who treats primarily cosmological illnesses has contributed to a neglect of those illnesses that are viewed by forest residents as treatable with pharmaceutical medicines, if such medicines cannot be readily obtained. This is not to suggest that *ombiasa* do not contribute substantially to health and healing in Madagascar, but that their contribution in this regard has diminished with the introduction of pharmaceutical medicines. As the availability of pharmaceutical medicines is curtailed, however, the role of the *ombiasa* in treating what many Westerners regard as biomedical disease[5] is not necessarily increasing. In addi-

---

4. These are my translations of the terms used to categorize illness among my informants (*aretina Zanahary* "illness of God," and *aretina antitra* "illness of the elderly, or aged.")

5. Throughout this book I refer to "Western" medicine in contrast to "indigenous" medicine, or to "biomedical disease" or biomedicine, in contrast to indigenous concepts of health and healing. This dichotomy is not necessarily the most precise characterization of cross-cultural healing systems, but reflects prevailing concepts in medical anthropology regarding the philosophical underpinnings of distinctive medical systems. Biomedicine is the medical system arising in the 18th century in Europe and America, which views disease as a biological or biochemical malfunction (Strathern and Stewart 1999:6), while indigenous medicine is a broad category reflecting the multiple explanations and beliefs concerning health and healing that are found in indigenous societies. Indigenous medicine includes not only cosmological beliefs, but also the use of plants, fauna, minerals, earth and water to heal. As such, indigenous medicine may in many respects be biologically efficacious, just as biomedicine may work hand-in-hand with cosmological views of healing

tion, rather than finding that increased poverty led to increased use of plant medicines, whether provided by indigenous healers or others, I found this to be true only of acute illnesses. Regarding chronic, long-term, illnesses, I found that increased poverty led to increased illness neglect.

Those most impoverished suffered from increasing illnesses of poverty, including severe malnutrition. Illnesses that were formerly treated by the traveling physician, or prior to him, Western-trained nurses and physicians (affiliated with colonial or post-colonial national healthcare available until the late 1980s in the nearby towns of Ranomafana or Ifanadiana), were, by the mid-1990's, often left untreated until they became so severe that they affected one's ability to work. These illnesses included scabies, venereal diseases, and respiratory infections. Whereas some acute conditions, such as malaria and serious respiratory infections, would continue to be treated with the plant medicines that had formerly been used in tandem with pharmaceutical medicines, the plant medicines were now used almost exclusively for these acute illnesses. But the use of plants alone was not viewed by many villagers as sufficient; illnesses frequently became so grave that the sick person could no longer function effectively within the society, and it was at this point that alternatives to plant medicines were more commonly sought, be they medicines of the pharmacy or of the *ombiasa*.

In the case of sick children, their mothers, rather than their fathers, often suffered the loss of work. Although informants indicated that mothers and fathers would both stay home and care for the children, it was rare for a father to do so. On the other hand, it was fathers who transported sick children to the hospital at Ranomafana, and thus they also lost work. If, however, there was an older female at home to care for sick children, then she would do so. As more older women were themselves pushed into wage labor or their workloads otherwise compounded, this childcare option was not always available.

At the same time that land-use and economic changes were causing many to become more poor and thus less healthy, those who were benefitting from the economic changes associated with conservation of the forests and privatization of the land, were in many cases able to continue purchasing antibiotics and Chloriquine (for treating malaria), as well as soap and food—resources that are essential to maintaining good health.

While most villagers endured severe health consequences associated with their intensified poverty, as well as illnesses associated with their trop-

as "God's will." Moreover, in using these dichotomies, I in no way intend to suggest that all indigenous people share the same thoughts on health and healing; as this study shows, they hold many diverse views on the subject, just as "Westerners" hold multiple, competing, and constantly changing views of medicine. This issue is discussed in more detail in the following chapter.

ical environment (e.g., malaria, hepatitis, and tuberculosis), they were struck by the irony that the very Westerners who they perceived — rightly or wrongly — to have cut off their supply of pharmaceutical medicines, were interested in their plant medicines, as environmental education and *sensibilisation*[6] programs have suggested.

Enter, the anthropologist. I was hardly the first researcher to arrive on the village threshold, begging for cooperation and promising abstract rewards. Indeed, I had selected the village for the very fact that it was one of the project's pilot villages, and as such, its residents had previously been subjected to numerous questionnaires, surveys, interviews and interventions. Among them had been an in-depth public health survey documenting the health status, nutritional intake, and daily activities of the residents (Kightlinger, et al. 1992). These findings were intended as baseline health data, from which future research could assess the impact of the park and project on resident's lives. Consequently, I was confident that my own research would contribute substantially toward this effort, and the previous health research, combined with the records of the visiting health team and with additional research concerning agricultural practices and environmental change, would provide me essential information with which to analyze relationships between health and environmental change from an ethnographic perspective.

But as happens with most research projects, the initial focus of my inquiry changed somewhat. In the course of my residency in the village, two social factors critically influenced my research methodology and findings. First, the presence of the national park project not only affected local lives, it affected nearly every facet of my research, as project administrators sought — and achieved — direct and indirect control of my research (discussed in more detail in the Epilogue). I was not without notice that such control was likely to ensue; indeed, every social scientist who had conducted research in the park region had indicated to me that they had been subjected to intense scrutiny by project administrators, pressured to produce findings consistent with project objectives, and in several instances expelled from the region or country when they displeased project administrators. And on a previous visit to the region in 1993, I witnessed the persecution of a female sociologist whose criticisms of the project were met with a lengthy inquiry into her sexuality and personal behavior; although the allegations levied against her were unfounded, the rumors they generated resulted in her departure from the island. As such, I initiated my research with great caution. I mistakenly believed, however, that by

---

6. The French term for environmental sensitivity programs, or "making one sensible," a term that continues to be employed by environmental NGO's, including the RNPP.

remaining relatively independent of the project, I would avoid such repression.

A second factor shaping my research was unrelated, at least directly, to such political issues. The village I selected was regarded by many as cursed. It was believed to be cursed because many of its residents were dying. During my fourteen month residency, eighteen people died—comprising roughly ten percent of the village's population of approximately 180 people.

The deaths were variously attributed to respiratory disorders, seizures, malnutrition, fevers, liver problems and ghost sickness. As every few weeks, or sometimes every day, another person died, suddenly or following an illness, I reflected more and more on whether or not the village had indeed been cursed. Standing outside a home filled with the wailing relatives and friends of one man suddenly dead in the middle of the night, the third that week, I felt a darkness engulf me as I began to faint—fearing I would be next. Were they indeed dying because some cosmological curse had struck this seemingly exotic corner of the globe—a cosmological force that I could not in my educated ignorance begin to comprehend? Or were they dying for some more mundane reason? Ten percent dead in just over a year suggested to me that either the ancestors were indeed displeased, or an environmental explanation was at hand. Of course, I did not dismiss the possibility, as many villagers suggested, that both explanations were true—the ancestors were displeased and so they sent this environmental curse upon them.

Given that there was a history of environmental, health, and economic data concerning this village having been gathered both before and after its establishment as a pilot village of the project, I believed that I had to bring the death rate to the attention of the project administrators, who were delegated, by the United States Agency for International Development, with responsibility for exploring the social ramifications of the recent social and environmental changes.

Clearly, the association between the deaths and the enclosure of the farming lands for biodiversity protection, as well as recent economic changes, were not necessarily causal nor even necessarily linked. But when there have been recently introduced environmental and economic changes, and a few years later there is an acceleration of what appear to be environmentally-related deaths among impoverished people, there might be a possible connection. Exploring such a connection was in keeping with the objectives of my research. At the very least, as a resident and guest of the village, I felt it my moral responsibility to seek help from those with access to health and economic data, and health and economic resources.

Unfortunately, calling attention to the high death rate, and seeking access to health documents and economic data, were regarded by my compatriots as not only outside the bounds of inquiry into "plants," but embarrassing and potentially subversive. My efforts to access data and address the health crisis I was witnessing, led to increasing concern among project administrators that my research, once of no interest to them, now required close supervision. The rigid surveillance of my research that I perceived to ensue, and the resistance of project officials to *any* social science inquiry in the southeastern forest region (regardless of distance from the park or relevance to the project) that the expatriate administration did not wholly control, prevented me from systematically examining whether there was indeed a causal relationship or other link between imposed environmental and social changes, and the escalating sickness and death in the region. Moreover, the controls exercised over my research illuminated for me the ways in which the scientific process itself is culturally conditioned. The questions that I was encouraged to ask, the questions I was discouraged from asking, and the data that were made available to me, as well as that which were withheld, all influenced the way that I perceived and analyzed the cultural context of environmental change and human health. It further influenced the conclusions that I have been able to present, limiting any findings regarding how the creation of the national park, or the development initiatives introduced in the region, have affected human health.

Nevertheless, I believe the story of the village, including the presence of an ethnographer herself deeply embedded in the political conflicts of the region, provides a telling portrait of a world gone wrong—one that multiple players desperately sought to keep going, each in differing ways and each toward differing ends. While the world in which we battled could hardly be characterized as a harmonious Eden before foreigners came along, this once imperfect system became impaired even further by both outsiders and insiders, all struggling for survival, if not dominance, as the forests receded from their grasp. And as struggles for power intensified, rather than diminished, local residents faced greater difficulties in reconciling their individual needs with the needs of their communities and the needs of the Malagasy state, and finally, with the international interests of conservation and globalization.

Not only did these circumstances shape my methodology and frame my research questions, they also helped to shape my theoretical perspective. While I set out to do a relatively conventional study in medical anthropology, I was not fully aware of the kinds of relationships that existed between health status of the residents of Ranotsara, and the rapidly changing economic circumstances brought about by the project and other factors. I was particularly unaware of the salience of the distinctive lineages in the village, and how economic changes and interventions would deepen this social divide and influence the meanings attached to the respective kinship ties.

I was also unsuspecting of how politicized these changes and the high death rate in Ranotsara were in the eyes of the project. Once I became aware of these relationships and processes, the focus and scope of my study broadened to include these factors at the same time that my ability to gain access to the data to examine them was curtailed and manipulated by the project administrators. In large part, this restriction of data was due to misunderstandings about the concerns of anthropology. Whereas anthropologists are increasingly pointing to the ways in which institutional and political structures underlie the disproportionately high levels of disease and malnutrition among the poor, people of color, and women, we are still regarded as specialists of the exotic; that is, as long as we focus on belief systems and curious taboos to understand illness and its treatment of 'the other,' we are regarded as "doing anthropology." But when we begin to question political and economic forces shaping morbidity and mortality among the poor, we are all too often regarded as venturing outside our discipline and not being anthropologists. And as Farmer (1999:248-260) has shown, anthropologists have also contributed to this bias, by emphasizing "cultural" factors over factors related to structural inequality that contribute to death and disease among the world's poorest people. Although I attempted to clarify the scope of anthropology to those who controlled the data I sought, my research was expected to focus on shamans and plant medicines exclusively.[7] Yet by restricting my access to information and people, the project administration provided me with the privilege of studying and experiencing the kinds of power relations which many anthropologists have suggested lie at the heart of cultural relations and contested resources.

In the following chapters, I return to further discussions and descriptions of the Ranomafana National Park Project, and I discuss the realities of life and death in Ranotsara, as contrasted to the public image conjured by project administrators and promoters, who contend that conservation of the forest is linked to improved health and well-being of forest residents. The actual benefits residents have received from the project, in exchange for relinquishing rights to the forest land, are discussed in terms of the health care they did and did not receive, their changing economic status, and how such changing economics shaped their society, their health and their access to health care.

The relationship between access to forest medicines and the changing forest environment, however, cannot be viewed solely as a relationship between village residents and the park project. The national park is central to the research setting and integral to the relationship between access to

---

7. Research proposals indicating that the research would include a political economy focus were submitted to the RNPP, ANGAP and the Ministry of Water and Forests. Research clearance was thereby granted, but I continued to be told by RNPP administrators that I was to study "plants."

health resources and the changing forest landscape. Moreover, the presence of the expatriate and national elite community in their roles as project managers and staff, provides a significant and provocative social context in which to understand contemporary social change in Ranotsara. Nonetheless, they represent physical and social components of a cultural complexity that includes multiple and competing interests within and beyond the village, extending from the households of Ranotsara to the national capital of Antananarivo, and the international comforts of the World Bank in Geneva.

While these places and players shape the transforming history of the forests of Ranotsara, and the health and medical spectrum of its people, how national and international processes affect local lives is not experienced by all villagers evenly. As I show in Chapter Six, the village is divided by two distinct lineages, with ancestry, rather than other cultural identities, having more to do with access to, and use of, resources. Moreover, the recent economic changes associated with agricultural liberalization, structural adjustment policies, and the penetration of conservation and development ideology, have further divided the village into a minority of land-owners (or controllers) and a majority of land laborers. These social divisions, and the changing organization of labor and society associated with them, provide the foundation for understanding the cultural context in which health and health care are manifest.

This study contextualizes the use of medicine within a model of culture in which culture is seen as active, changing, and contested, comprising multiple individual experiences that converge, diverge, coincide, and contradict. While shared interests may be apparent when a society is positioned against the interests of the state or other outside agents, closer scrutiny reveals that, encroaching forces of the state aside, at the local level various components of the medical system can be understood as contested resources. These resources are differentially accessed in terms of power relations at multiple social levels, relations which are understood as arising from both the changing organization of labor (related to the penetration of capitalism in the form of privatized land, a greater reliance on the market economy, imposed changes in the mode of subsistence), and from a history of shifting identities tied to one's ancestry.

The geographical scale of a village-level study provides insights into the use of medicines in a tropical forest community, where power relations are becoming increasingly differentiated within a single generation. While representing a single year in a single community, such insights do permit one to draw conclusions about forest medicine use in a broader context. The very personal stories which unfold illuminate the reality of forest farmers as being variable, unique, and shaped by both social and personal experience. As such, to reduce a group of people to their purported "culture" provides an inaccurate portrait of their lives, as well as that of others categorically placed within the bounds of a particular culture. This is not to suggest that an understanding of culture is by its very nature misleading or false (indeed, I argue that understanding how culture shapes one's world view is essential to understanding human behavior). I suggest, instead, that culture should be understood in terms of the differences and changes which create it, and the meanings which are imposed upon such differences and changes.

Clarifying the "Cultural" Context of Environmental Change

In much public health research, as well as in ethnobotanical studies and in the development literature (where the policy implications of public health and ethnobotanical research are often manifest), the intersections of "culture" and the natural world have been approached in a near cavalier fashion. Development planners often remain limited in their concepts of how environmental change is related to culture by late-nineteenth century views of culture as an undifferentiated "thing" to be defined and manipulated in order to bring its members into the modern world. The social forces by which culture is created are often obscured by myopic views of culture as inseparable from unchanging "traditions."

Moreover, those social forces that are identified as "cultural," may be limited to observations of the features and practices that are obvious and outstanding to the observer. The closer one's material world, economic system, language, and belief system correspond to that of the (Western) observer, the less likely these features and practices will be deemed "cultural," or in need of change. Conversely, where practices and beliefs are deemed to be different, they are more likely to be judged as "cultural" phenomena.

As Abu-Lughod (1991) notes, culture is a conceptual tool used to create 'the other.' In so doing, differences cast as cultural may be so rigidly fixed in the mind of the observer that they appear innate, or racial. Such casting of social forces and practices as cultural is particularly salient to understandings of health and environmental change in Madagascar, where "ethnicity" has been conjured by project planners and the state to explain forest degradation, economic status, and agricultural practices. By defining ethnicity as the most important social variable determining resource use, the state and the project are operating under perversely distorted concepts of community and culture that only deepen the chasm between Western conservationists and local residents. This chasm is made all the more unbridgeable, as the forest is literally and conceptually treated as a naturally bounded "ecosystem" separate from the humans that inhabit and create it.

As discussed in more detail throughout this book, the Ranomafana National Park Project presumed local "culture" to be the determining factor in how the environment was used and what people believed and practiced. These ideas were largely the outcome of sloppy reading of the ethnography in the region, in which project administrators conflated "culture" with both ethnicity and land-use practices. Much of the social research in the region (e.g. Ferraro 1994; Harrison 1992; Kottak 1980) has tended toward a theoretical orientation of environmental determinism or cultural materialism. Cultural materialism, arising from the early cultural ecology studies of Julian Steward and developed by his student, Marvin Harris, focuses on

> the interaction between behavior and environment as mediated by the human organism and its cultural apparatus. It does so as an order of priority with the prediction that group structure and ideology are responsive to these classes of material conditions (Harris 1968: 659).

Cultural materialism suggests that certain cultural features will be selected for or against so that, over time, culture does change, but this change is toward greater adaptation to the environment, in much the same way as natural selection works to select for certain adaptive physical traits. It does not, however, suggest an identifiable direction, but remains, instead, opportunistic (Harris 1999).

Harris (1999) suggested that cultural materialism rests on the theory that the infrastructure[8], or in this case, mode of subsistence, is a primary determinant of cultural traits.

> The principle of the primacy of infrastructure holds that innovations that arise in the infrastructural sector are likely to be preserved and propagated if they enhance the efficiency of the productive and reproductive processes that sustain health and well-being and that satisfy basic human biopsychological needs and drives (Harris 1999:142).

The cultural materialist perspective has been used to explain land-use practices in Madagascar through Kottak's (1971a; 1971b; 1980) ethnographic studies of the highland Betsileo. Kottak, a student of Harris, sug-

---

8. Harris (1992:297) defined "infrastructure" as "technological, economic, demographic, and environmental activities and conditions directly related to sustaining health and well-being through the social control of production and reproduction."

gested that culture change in Madagascar can be understood as Malagasy populations adapting to their differing environments. To summarize Kottak's argument, for those living in the steep, forested hills, swidden rice farming, or *tavy*, has been an efficient mode of production. For those living in flatter regions, irrigated agriculture has been more efficient. Hence, those living in the plateau regions who were assigned to the administrative division "Betsileo" in the 18th century, had a history of irrigated agriculture. For those living in the forested region, who termed themselves "Tanala" or People of the Forest, *tavy* was an adaptive subsistence strategy. As "Betsileo" moved to the forested hills, they taught the forest residents techniques of irrigated agriculture, and at the same time, they learned techniques in swidden horticulture.

In this view, changing subsistence patterns (or *infrastructure*) are the catalyst to cultural change. Project administrators interpreted these views to suggest that irrigated agriculture was a more efficient form of subsistence than swidden, and imposed a unilineal evolutionary framework on their own ideas of social change (quite distinct from the intent of Steward's cultural ecology or Harris' cultural materialism). Hence, it was believed by policy makers and project administrators that irrigated agriculture is more progressive than swidden agriculture, and this progression was assumed to be based on greater efficiency and production, with no meaningful measure of whether or not such efficiency or production was actually realized by those making the shift from swidden horticulture to irrigated agriculture.

While cultural materialism does explain current practices and views in a general sense, and lends a useful perspective to understandings of how the agricultural system, economic systems, and various forms of social organization interrelate, it does not fully account for the diversity of behaviors and views among local residents. Harris (1999) addressed concerns that cultural materialism does not account for separate and conflicting interests.

> In the presence of groups with conflicting interests, selection for or against innovations depends on the relative power that each group can exert on behalf of its own interests. Unlike most Marxian treatments of this problem, however, cultural materialism recognizes the occurrence of innovations that simultaneously benefit both subordinate and superordinate groups. In stratified societies, substantial changes in any sector generally occur only when they benefit the superordinate groups (classes, genders, ethnicities) to some extent; but this does not mean that the subordinate groups do not benefit, if generally to a lesser degree, from the same innovations (Harris 1999:143).

Cultural materialism thus presents a "trickle-down" theory of cultural change, in which changes occur only to the extent that they benefit those in power, but that to a greater or lesser extent those with lesser power will also benefit. What remains unexplained is that to a greater extent, in many cases, those with lesser power are significantly harmed. For large sectors of the population, cultural innovations may well be maladaptive. Harris (1999) contended that cultural materialism does indeed acknowledge the maladaptive nature of certain features, but that if a cultural feature is truly maladaptive for everyone, it will not be selected for. On the other hand, if the feature is adaptive for certain groups in power, such as slavery or colonialism, it will persist despite the fact that it is maladaptive for the majority, at least until it is no longer adaptive for the group in power. This view remains unsatisfactory because it does not explain how a feature that is maladaptive for the majority of the group can be maintained nor how it can be viewed as adaptive in a general sense, a presumption that is necessary if one is to accept cultural materialist explanations of culture change. Moreover, it does not allow for the rich variety in interpretive aspects of culture, that is, how multiple and often conflicting meanings are given to specific cultural features, regardless of their adaptive or maladaptive nature. How, for example, can one explain the differing meanings of ancestry in the community of Ranotsara, where, as explained in Chapter Six, one's descent can simultaneously be viewed as a source of shame and a source of pride?

An alternative perspective can be gleaned from arguments raised by Eleanor Burke Leacock (1982), who suggested that changes in the organization of labor characteristic of the shift to capitalist modes of production lead to changes in how groups compete for labor and resources. She was particularly concerned with exploring the historical context of cultural change, finding such change more closely related to changes in the organization of labor than in the mode of subsistence. Moreover, these changes lead to the subordination of certain groups, and their political subordination enables cultural practices that may well be maladaptive to persist.

But by prioritizing science over history, as conservationists have done, rather than understanding that ecologies have histories, it becomes impossible to understand how local populations have lived with their environments. Chase (1986), for example, has shown how Yellowstone National Park was mismanaged for decades, and with profound repercussions to the ecology of the area, by a failure to incorporate the history of Native American land use practices in the region. Instead, by presuming Native Americans had no history in the region, or that any history they might have had was insignificant, the ways in which Native Americans both protected and destroyed the region, were not incorporated into "scientific" understandings of the artificially-bounded ecosystem.

Finally, there is another important consideration regarding how cultural concepts are applied to understanding the relationships between health and the environment. As Foucault (1979:271) has observed regarding penal institutions, social problems become removed from the realm of politics and placed in the realm of technology as the prison system combines coercive regulations with scientific propositions, social effects, and "invincible utopias." Social problems are no longer understood as *political* problems, but are instead regarded as *technological* problems, requiring technological, or scientific, solutions.

The theoretical perspectives that I build upon draw out the anthropological context of forest healing to illuminate the social and political dimensions of the scientific process. It shows that culture is alive—that those who become sick and die, those who gather leaves and bark for healing illnesses, those who walk across bridges and hills to reach pharmacies to buy antibiotics for their children—are people with names; they are not faceless tribal members blindly pledging allegiance to tradition. They are instead creators, by creating new practices that may or may not be consistent with "cultural traditions."

In this study, I do not attempt to explain what is causing forest loss in southeastern Madagascar, although I do show how historical changes have contributed to this loss. What I explain, instead, is how the "tradition" of *tavy* is tied to a changing society and changing forest landscape. Further, I show how cultural "identities" are perceived by both outsiders, who make and enforce policy, and by insiders, those who live in the forested hills and are judged "ethnic."

In a study of access to health resources in an environment in which U.S. and global interests have imposed drastic measures limiting access to forest resources (by prohibiting access to the forest), one could indeed easily fall prey to political and economic reductionism by claiming the seizure of ancestral lands has caused the community to become impoverished, thereby leading to illness. In order to avoid the economic reductionism that often accompanies analyses of power relations, some political ecologists have cautioned against regarding social and environmental change as exclusively outcomes of capitalism. Bryant (1992:13) cites Blaikie (1989) on this point:

> any attempt to attribute desertification to "natural forces" other than the penetration of capitalism is written off in some quarters as merely a bourgeois red herring. This is a simplistic and unnecessary polarisation since it is the dialectic between environmental and social change which must provide the context in which land degradation is discussed.

In an effort to avoid such reductionism, I show how the relationship between access to medicines and access to the forest is mediated by state and local-level dynamics interacting with international policies. In many ways, the creation of the national park and the way in which it has been managed have indeed contributed significantly to economic and social stratification (Hanson 1997), thereby enriching a minority, who in turn control agricultural and economic resources available to the majority.

In many other ways, however, despite the influx of international wealth to facilitate changes in resource management, the international community has had very little direct impact in the way that the forest is used, health resources are accessed, and residents' lives are affected. National and local histories and policies have far more salience in the lives of most of the residents than has the multi-million-dollar-funded Ranomafana National Park Project (cf. Ferguson 1994). The ramifications of an international conservation and development project on the economic status or world views of most people living in Ranotsara are so abstract that it is no more understandable to a local forest farmer than it is to a project administrator. Nonetheless, as I will show, international powers (both colonial and post-colonial) that have imposed environmental policies on residents, and the disproportionate distribution of funds and agricultural assistance in the region, *have* had an impact on local power relations. At the same time, local level dynamics, rooted in a history of domestic slavery, forbidden marriages, and contested claims to land and power, have also contributed to contemporary social inequalities and conflicts that now influence who benefits and who loses from environmental and economic change. These changing and differing interests have consequently shaped the relationships between access to health resources and access to forest resources. Such local-level outcomes underscore the problems of applying a standard model of conservation and development to diverse societies without taking into account that such policies will be received, resisted, and incorporated in unique and unexpected ways.

Political Ecology of Health

In this study, I draw on what I term a "political ecology of health perspective." While there have been earlier efforts to present a "political ecology of health" position (e.g. Baer 1996; Gruenbaum 1996; Leatherman 1996), efforts which have successfully extended critical medical anthropology to include ecological factors, they have not had much basis in political ecology analyses. For example, Baer (1996:452) describes how he views political ecology:

> Like critical medical anthropology, contemporary political economy has at best given passing consideration to environmental factors. However, neo-Marxist and other radical scholars are at-

tempting to integrate ecological considerations into their analyses of various types of societies. Such endeavors have been referred to as the "political economy of ecology" (O'Connor 1989), "eco-Marxism" (Benton 1989; DeLeague 1989; Grundman 1991; Raskin and Bernow 1991), "eco-socialism" (Pepper 1993; Ryle 1988), "radical ecology" (Merchant 1992), "socialist ecology," and "social ecology." Much of the interest in what I simply term "political ecology" stems from Green politics in Europe, particularly Germany, and has been inspired by the work of neo-Marxist scholars such as Andre Gorz (1980) and Rudolf Bahro (1982) and ecoanarchist Murray Bookchin (1989).

This definition provides a useful summary of those scholars who have addressed environmental and social issues, but in so doing, it groups an extensive range of theories and methodologies, and does not include those scholars who have been in the forefront of framing an explicitly political ecology perspective (e.g. Blaikie and Brookfield 1987; Bryant 1992; Bryant and Bailey 1997; Watts 1989). Moreover, while Baer's summary of political *economy* approaches to the environment illuminates scholarship that is based on critical perspectives of the study of humans and their environments, his definition fails to recognize that a more complex situation prevails. Rather than simply being an outgrowth of Green politics in Europe, political *ecology* focuses on specific methods and levels of analysis aimed at explicating the connections among local, national and international processes related to ecological change, while at the same time illuminating how society and environment are differentially experienced by specific social groups. Political ecology also focuses on how those who live within an environment are not only affected by ecological change, but also actively fashion and form it. As such, environmental change is not just something that people passively experience, but it is also something that they construct.

Baer's comments do, however, suggest a recognition of the need for critical medical anthropologists to pay greater attention to the role of the environment in shaping health. Nonetheless, there remains a need to delve deeper into the literature of "political ecology" to draw out how such theorists have explored the ways in which differing levels of power interact with social and environmental change. Moreover, just as medical anthropologists have used the term "political ecology" while failing to incorporate theoretical perspectives from political ecology into their analyses, political ecologists have given little attention to the sphere of health, viewing indigenous medical systems as homogenous, and disease as exclusively a biological process. How people variously experience sickness, how indigenous classifications of disease are shaped by changing environments, how medical resources are differently interpreted — as well as accessed — by local populations, and how people interpret the relationship between their environments and their health — remain to be understood by political ecologists examining the relationships between ecology and health. By bridging political ecology with the political economy of health, and in so doing, incorporating interpretive analyses of health and ecology, better understandings of local-level strategies to access the resources of health become possible (e.g. Ennis McMillan 2001).

As anthropologists begin to address these issues in regard to the environmental health nexus, a similar critique is emerging in the discipline of geography. The failure of political ecologists to address issues of health, and of medical geographers to address issues of inequality, has been noted by Mayer (1996; 2000) who advocates a political ecology of disease framework by which to analyze social processes shaping disease ecology (1996). He proposes that a political ecology of disease approach must show how large-scale political, social and economic processes influence local practices and disease ecology, and argues that the local contexts of disease must be understood and related to the macro-dimensions of political economy. By exploring the interconnections of differing scales, Mayer suggests, patterns of disease ecology will be illuminated in ways which conventional approaches to the intersections of health and disease have failed to do.

> Disease ecology, so basic to medical geography and epidemiology, is also a powerful approach to understanding disease emergence and resurgence (May 1958; Meade 1976). Many changes that are relevant to understanding emerging and resurgent diseases are due to political and economic power at a variety of scales, ranging from the transnational down to the household and individual levels. Some, or even much of this power is influenced by which groups control decisions over land use. This, in turn, influences the relationships of people and the environment. This is a basic principle of political ecology which has received some attention in the geography of health and disease (Mayer 1996), and has been used increasingly in understanding the consequences of human-environment interactions (Mayer 2000:938).

Building on these ongoing efforts to integrate political ecology with the social context of health and disease, I use the term "political ecology of health" to refer to multiple levels of well-being, illness, and disease. In this way, health is to be understood as an experiential state, which may or may not include biomedical concepts of disease. As this study will show, however, I regard the prevalence of (biomedically-defined) disease in developing countries as a critical social issue which the promotion of "natural" medicines as healing agents fails to address; a political ecology of disease approach is therefore compelling.

Toward such an understanding of the political ecology of health and disease, I examine ways in which historical and contemporary interventions aimed at controlling land and society have penetrated the body through illness, disease, and death. In the tradition of political ecology, I focus not only on how people have been affected by the political economy of the region, but also on how they have exercised their own wills to survive. One strategy toward survival has been through the quest for medicine. I examine medicines as *resources* of the forest, and explore the differing strategies to obtain these resources by those who live in the forest. Such an examination requires an understanding of forest medicines as *those substances perceived and used by forest residents as healing substances*. This definition includes pharmaceutical medicines, as much as it does plants or other substances. It does not necessitate that the substance be found in the forest; rather it regards forest medicines as those medicines used by people living in forest communities. As such, medicines symbolize the power of the ancestors (whose knowledge of plant use has been passed through generations, and who have bestowed on certain plants healing properties), but also the power of the outside world (to restore health and fend off death and disease). Further, by the very nature of such an examination of medicines as resources, and thereby *property*, the salience of *access* to health resources is illuminated—which means understanding economic differentiation, social differences, and environmental change in the shaping of resource use.

I also incorporate concepts from political ecology regarding social stratification as not merely a bi-product of capitalism. As I present in Chapter Five, pre-capitalist state formation contributed to social hierarchies in Madagascar; these hierarchies, in turn, have shaped contemporary power relations at the local level. Further, in my discussions of social stratification as it is related to the more recent penetration of capitalism, I build on Morgan's (1984) call to treat capitalism in terms of the means of production, including land, labor, capital, and technology. By exploring class in relation to means of production, rather than "the market," one can better examine the uneven ways that capitalism affects people, and the ways that people actively engage or resist it.

Finally, I emphasize that indigenous knowledge is not uniform within a culture (Warren 1997). Different people have different knowledge domains, and these multiple ways of knowing shape health and health care differently for different people, as well as contribute to medical pluralism. An understanding of the complexity of indigenous knowledge domains as they converge with Western knowledge domains, contributes to an analysis of forest medicines in the context of social and environmental change.

Issues Raised in the Presentation of People

This study is organized as a story of a land and people. It is couched in history because it is impossible to understand the story otherwise. It is contrasted to policy—particularly international environmental and economic policies that penetrate the far reaches of the forest in search of genetic material for "global" commodification, and protection of "pristine ecosystems" for Western science and tourism.

But in presenting history and policy, I do so by recurrently engaging the voices of the villagers who hosted my stay. The specific quotes are taken from notes of events and conversations. In some cases, in order to make particular dialogues and anecdotes memorable, and to make the people more real to the reader, I elaborate on the discourse from memory. Although a verbal exchange may be embellished to provide more authenticity, the explanation or point reported is taken from notes or tape-recorded interviews. In cases in which I attribute a particular position to a particular institutional representative, I indicate by citation that my information was derived from direct, personal communication with that person.

I have used pseudonyms throughout the book, and have done so in order to protect the anonymity of my informants in accordance with my university agreement regarding the rights of human subjects. Nonetheless, I am not entirely comfortable with this decision, because most of the informants with whom I lived and studied regarded themselves as individuals whose views were important, if continually ignored. By failing to use their own names, it may appear that I am rendering them more anonymous than they prefer, but it is a dilemma I cannot easily resolve. For administrators of the Ranomafana National Park, I use neither names nor pseudonyms. I have used, instead, professional titles only, translated into English. My reason for choosing this route is that they were operating, albeit as individuals with unique personalities and psychologies, as institutional representatives, and it would matter little who wore these hats. The names of all researchers, however, are real.

While Ranotsara is a pseudonym, all other place names are real, as is the Ranomafana National Park. All institutions referred to are real and referred to by their given names or acronyms; to have used pseudonyms would have made it impossible to draw upon institutional documents to support my claims.

The use of tense is always problematic in ethnography. To use the past tense implies that things *were*, that people *were*, that the people one writes about have ceased being with the departure of the ethnographer. On the other hand, to use the present tense implies that things have not changed since the departure of the ethnographer, when in fact, lives have continued and changes have unfolded. What was true during the period of fieldwork may not be true by the time the ethnography is written.

I cannot solve the problem of tense, I can only choose that which suits the narrative best. In this case, when speaking of specific events, I use the past tense, because they did happen. But when providing ethnographic or political detail, I use the present tense unless I know the situation has changed. The choice to do so does not imply that changes have not occurred, but indicates only that to the best of my knowledge, the situation probably remains much the same.[9]

Regarding my own role in the ethnography, I have chosen to include my presence, because it did indeed have a significant impact in the village. I introduced material objects to the village which had previously been absent, or in some cases totally unknown. I brought with me various pharmaceutical medicines. I introduced my own ideas and politics by way of daily discussions with others concerning their ideas and politics. To have concealed my views while eliciting their own would have been deceptive and furthered our differences. I also brought into the community a micro-economy by providing jobs and loans. No matter how "objectively" I tried to draw out class inequalities and tensions, there was no escaping the fact that I certainly reproduced class inequality by the glaring gap between my access to resources and those of the people with whom I lived. Although I tried to learn about and follow as much as I could their way of living, and was often affectionately labeled "Tanala," with newly accomplished skills or understandings, I know that I remained a privileged white outsider in many people's eyes.

Another issue which I feel it necessary to address is the role of research assistants in this project. When I began my fieldwork, I employed a research assistant who helped me to negotiate unfamiliar cultural terrain, handle multiple details associated with relocating and settling in a village, and interpreting the language. His assistance was, initially, invaluable to me, but it was not without its shortcomings. As most anthropologists have discovered, the use of a research assistant for translation may make the initial work easier, but dependence on another slows the anthropologist in mastering the language. Moreover, he was formally educated, middle class, and from an urban area rather distant from the site. These factors contributed to some hesitancy on the part of informants to disclose certain information, and his own biases regarding *andevo* [slave] and "Tanala" identities probably influenced his interpretations. Finally, prior to my hiring

---

9. I have made every effort possible to substantiate where changes have taken place, but communication with both the village and the project have been limited since my departure due to the relative isolation of the village and the resistance of project personnel to this research project.

him, he was affiliated with the Ranomafana National Park Project as a tourist guide; as the tension between myself and the project deepened, and the project offered him permanent employment and other benefits, and regularly solicited information from him regarding me and the research, it became necessary that I work independent of a research assistant. In so doing, I discovered that working on my own enabled me to communicate without assistance, and to discover histories, ideas, and meanings that had formerly either been concealed, or filtered through another's subjectivity. At the same time, the loss of my research assistant revealed the many ways in which working with another had strengthened my work. For example, he provided me with insights and information regarding men that I had not otherwise gained, as I worked primarily with women. In addition, the continual discussions we had shared had helped me to articulate and develop my own ideas. While others subsequently assisted me in small parts of the research, I ceased relying on full-time assistance for the last six months of the project.

What follows, then, is the story of what I learned, never having shaken the role of material privilege into which I was born, and never having found some secret passage into "Tanala culture," revealing hidden mysteries of the Other. This is a very Western story, after all.

Chapter 2

The Anthropology of Forest Medicine Use

In most of the popular literature and discourse on the "forest" and "medicines," as well as in health and conservation policies, forest medicines are inevitably perceived as plants beneficial to humankind (e.g. David 1997; Plotkin 1993). Indeed, the role plants and other botanical resources play in the health and well-being of humans is indisputable. But beyond the immediate perceptions one may form regarding the contribution botany makes to society, there remain more subtle, and more complex, dimensions to this relationship. To understand this relationship in greater depth, one must consider the ways in which public perceptions of the relationship between forest medicines and society have been shaped by both academic and commercial concerns.

There are two primary ways that forest medicines or medicinal plants are viewed by those who do not live in the forest (whom I term "outsiders"). One view regards forest medicines as resources to be commodified. As the multinational pharmaceutical industry expands its drug marketing globally, the commodification of tropical resources by capitalist enterprises also accelerates. With this expansion of the profit-oriented medicine industry, the concept of "traditional" has been reduced to that which is of little or no economic value to the Western world.

At the same time, ecologists and ethnobotanists present a second view. In the name of biodiversity and as a strategy and goal of sustainable development, they call for researching and preserving traditional medicines, and the indigenous knowledge systems concerning their use.

> The use of natural plant-derived medicines is perhaps the only sustainable form of medicine. It can foster a greater consciousness of the value of biodiversity while offering appropriate medicines for the developing and industrialized world and high-value crops for worldwide production. Botanical medicines are experiencing a meteoric rise in popularity worldwide, especially in the United States and Europe. The increased use of herbs for health can help save the environment, but this increased demand can also destroy local ecosystems and push threatened

plants to the brink of extinction. The key to achieving the positive potential of the natural health care movement is environmentally and socially conscious development and sustainable production of the botanical raw materials which feed this rapidly growing business (McCaleb 1997:221).

Warren (1997) indicated that research on the medicinal properties of plants is integrally linked to sustainability of environmental development through a focus on indigenous knowledge. Indigenous knowledge, he argued, is an important national resource; by recognizing intellectual property rights to profits from medicinal plants, and by including those knowledgeable as participants in the commodification and marketing of plants, medicinal plants become a key symbol to sustainability.

This focus on the preservation of biodiversity as a morally righteous objective has indeed been seized by the pharmaceutical industry seeking Third World resources for First World drugs. Their focus on "traditional" medicine has two objectives. One, to gain knowledge about the unknown medical system in order to appropriate both the knowledge and the resources for Western profit, and two, to gain knowledge about the unknown medical system in order to tap new markets for Western drugs. This knowledge and these resources thus obtained become "Western," whereas what is left behind as of no use, or what remains undiscovered by Western researchers or unfamiliar to them, is "traditional." This dichotomized ideology presumes that there is no tradition in Western allopathic medicine, nor anything modern in indigenous medicines.

To bridge this gap, some medical anthropologists have called for more attention to medical pluralism, as opposed to studies of medical "systems." While Stoner (1986) has charged that the "medical systems" have become dichotomized as "folk" or "modern," ignoring the multiple forms of medicine that practitioners employ to heal the sick, Comaroff (1983) and Stoner (1986) have critiqued the concept of medical system itself for the ethnocentric bias inherent in separating the medical from other social dimensions. Comaroff charges that the scientific quest for categories (within the medical system) is itself ethnocentric in that it presumes such categories to exist, and that the distinction of various social domains, such as religious, economic, or medical, are recognized as separate domains among the people whose medical system is studied by the ethnographer.

Baer, Singer and Susser (1997) suggest that medical pluralism is not indigenous to pre-state societies, but is instead, directly associated with increasing social stratification. They indicate that the role of shaman is primary to the dyadic core (healer-patient relationship) in simple preindustrial societies, whereas in horticultural societies one finds multiple specialists utilizing varying components of the folk medical system. In industrial societies, the authors suggest, the biomedical physician dominates a myriad of medical systems. They further contend that the concept of medical pluralism is perhaps better understood as medical dominative systems, in which biomedicine dominates all other systems.

While not disputing the association between increasing levels of social stratification and increasing medical specialization, I would suggest that this view reifies in some respects the folk/modern dichotomy by its reliance on subsistence strategies as boundaries separating "simple preindustrialm" foraging, horticultural, and state industrial societies. In reality, multiple subsistence strategies are practiced in all societies and all societies have been incorporated into states. Although certain subsistence strategies may predominate in societies, this does not necessarily mean that they are uniformly practiced by all community members. In this book, I show how a society characterized as both horticultural and agricultural is tied to the market and tied to the state, and its members engage in multiple subsistence strategies from foraging to irrigated agriculture; these practices, in turn, affect their health and access to medicines in different ways. To classify them as practitioners of folk and/or modern medicine, as I show in later chapters they have been, is as misleading as classifying them as swidden *or* irrigated rice agriculturalists. Their society has, nonetheless, changed significantly as wage labor becomes far more central to the economic base, at the same time the society resists efforts by outsiders to abandon foraging and horticultural practices in favor of irrigated agriculture. In other words, while the organization of labor is rapidly changing, the mode of subsistence is changing at a much slower pace. The increasing social stratification in the Ranomafana region is more closely related to the changing *structure* of the economy than it is to the mode of subsistence, or infrastructure. It is this changing economic base that is contributing to medical pluralism and inequalities in health and well-being, rather than the shift to irrigated agriculture per se.[1] These ideas are discussed in greater depth in the chapters which follow.

Biomedicine may well predominate in stratified societies, in that it is more desirable for certain people in the treatment of certain disorders, but

---

1. The changes in the economic base, however, act upon the mode of subsistence by limiting the labor available for some people to engage in horticultural practices, at the same time that it increases the labor available to others for expanding horticultural practices. With limited labor for either horticulture or agriculture, foraging increases for some people, but diminishes for others. The uneven ways in which these social changes are adaptive for some and maladaptive for others is central to an understanding of how the prevailing environmental policies of the Ranomafana National Park Project presumed cultural and social change to be predictable and progressive, in direct contrast to the cultural history of the region. These issues are discussed further in Chapters Four and Five.

I would argue that it does not always predominate. Likewise, while an emphasis on the hegemonic influence of biomedicine, particularly with regard to the commodification and distribution of pharmaceuticals, is imperative to understanding how biomedicine is incorporated into post-colonial societies and viewed by community members, such an emphasis can obscure an equally imperative emphasis on how biomedicine is often superior to plant medicine in treating many critical health issues—notwithstanding the fact that it is often injurious as well. It is for this reason that the World Health Organization (1988) has called for the equitable distribution of essential medicines throughout the globe.

Nonetheless, distinctions of "folk" and "modern" continue to be routinely employed by physicians and anthropologists alike, particularly in the study of medicines. van der Geest and Whyte (1988:10,11) have alluded to this problem:

> In situations of pharmaceutical pluralism, terms like "traditional" and "modern," "indigenous" and "Western" medicines are almost unavoidable. So are the quotation marks around these terms. There is an uncomfortable sense that they are misleading, since the pluralistic context transforms both imported and native medicines. Thus we find "modern" medicines being distributed by "traditional" healers and utilized in ways never imagined by the manufacturers. Penicillin may become an ancient Ayurvedic medicine. And we see "indigenous" medicine being manufactured on an enormous scale advertised on television, and exported to other countries. Genuine *jamu* from Indonesia can be purchased in Europe. The nuances involved here may serve to remind us once more of the care needed in the use of terms like traditional and Western medicine.

Concepts of "traditional" medicine are not just imposed on indigenous societies by outsiders from the Western world. They are just as likely to be perpetuated by outsiders from within post-colonial nations—that is, urban-based, Western-educated elite. Feierman (1985) suggests that there is an assumption in the medical anthropology research that "traditional" African medicine is something that "traditional" Africans do. This assumption is facilitated, in part, by the social status of those Africans who write about African medicine. Feierman points out that focusing on the competition between popular and biomedicine draws attention away from more critical questions, such as how are social costs distributed, what is the relationship between production and health, and how do social changes pattern health and disease?

Despite the convenience of distinguishing between traditional and Western medicine, and despite the seeming contrast between the domains, it is important to explore the political and economic forces that shape any concept of "medicine." In so doing, it becomes apparent that regardless of whether a medicine is found in the backyard or in a child-resistant plastic bottle, medicines are resources, and as resources, distinguishing them according to their material form may not tell as much about the person taking them as does distinguishing them in terms of their political and economic form.

> Time, space, matter, cause, relation, human nature, and society itself are social products created by man just as are the different types of tools, farming systems, clothes, houses, monuments, languages, myths, and so on, that mankind has produced since the dawn of human life. But to their participants, all cultures tend to present these categories as if they were not social products but elementary and immutable things. As soon as such categories are defined as natural, rather than social products, epistemology itself acts to conceal understanding of the social order. Our experience, our understanding, our explanations—all serve merely to ratify the conventions that sustain our sense of reality unless we appreciate the extent to which the basic 'building blocks' of our experienced and sensed reality are not natural but social constructions (Taussig 1980:4).

Nonetheless, the political and economic forms of medicine used by forest residents are rarely addressed by those who study them, except to the extent they are presumed to be profitable. This is because a second view many bring to the study of forest medicines is deeply embedded in Western views of what constitute such medicines. This is the view that forest medicines—primarily conceptualized as plant medicines—are natural healing agents from the forest's rich cornucopia of biodiversity. They are, as such, "good things," "natural," and potentially enriching both in terms of health and wealth.

> A growing segment of the public believes that herbal medicines and other alternatives are safer, possibly more effective, more natural, and more in harmony with a lifestyle that promotes self-care, individual responsibility, freedom of choice, and "holistic" thinking. A part of this too is the belief that a return to more natural therapies is a return to the time in which our medicines, like our foods, came from the earth, and the use of these natural substances is more in harmony with our natural surroundings (McCaleb 1997:228,229).

The view that forest medicines are medicinal plants and medicinal plants are by their very nature "natural," and "good," comes primarily from studies in ethnobotany and the recent popularization of ethnobotanical research in tropical forests (e.g. Davis 1985; Plotkin 1993). Three major themes have prevailed in this literature regarding the relationship between tropical forests and indigenous medicines. The first theme is that tropical forests are home to countless health resources — specifically, medicinal plants used by forest people for treating diseases and wounds, as well as providing nutrition. A classic example of the "global" value of tropical forest plants is Madagascar's Rosy Periwinkle. The Rosy Periwinkle is used indigenously to treat diabetes; discovered by Western scientists to be an effective treatment for childhood leukemia, it is frequently used as an example of the potential medical and economic value of tropical forest plants, suggesting that there are untold other plant species which can aid in the treatment of other cancers, heart disease and AIDS.[2]

A second theme which is an important concern to Western scientists and many environmentalists is that as forests are destroyed, indigenous communities, as well as the Western scientific community, may lose medicines. This line of intellectual query ignores the economic benefit forest residents may receive from burning the forest, leading to health benefits which in many circumstances may offset the loss of medicine. Consequently, the local context in which forest cover is intentionally cleared must be considered along with ethnographic inquiry into how medicines are used by forest residents. Without such ethnographic understanding, the extent to which the loss of plant medicines affects those who live in the forest is not clear. More attention has been drawn to the potential "global" loss of medicines — that is, the loss to Western medicine and pharmaceutical corporations — that deforestation might cause, than to how loss of forest diversity is or is not associated with the loss of medicines for forest residents.

A third theme is that increased population pressure leads to increased deforestation of the tropics; as forest residents increase swidden agriculture on a limited land base, they encroach on old growth rainforests. This theme is advanced by many conservation and development planners who are concerned with halting the destruction of tropical forests, and is central to the environmental and health policies of the World Bank and the United States Agency for International Development. This view holds that if women who live and work in tropical forests adopt family planning practices, and have access to improved prenatal and infant health care, forest populations will decrease, and forest residents will no longer need to clear more forested land. This view focuses more on how the health of people affects

---

2. Plotkin (1993) points out that the two drugs developed from the alkaloids of the Rosy Periwinkle led to annual sales of over $100 million, with no money being returned to Madagascar, the country of origin.

the health of the forest, presuming as well that what is good for the forest (conservation) is good for its inhabitants. Conservation planners and ethnobotanists consequently are concerned with conserving the forest in order to preserve plant species (e.g. Middleton, O'Keefe and Moyo 1993), with exploring shared indigenous knowledge systems of how local forest products are used by healing specialists (e.g. Naranjo 1995), and with investigating the cultural roles that plants play in indigenous communities (e.g. Alcorn 1995).

To persuade local forest communities of these "scientific" needs, environmental organizations often appeal to local communities to support conservation objectives by suggesting there is potential profit in local forest medicines. They often suggest that everyone will benefit if plants found to be of value to Westerners — either for medicines, perfumes, or beauty creams — can be marketed nationally or internationally.

> As countries like Cameroon begin to see the economic value of the medicinal plants in their forests, they can better appreciate the foolishness of clear-cutting those forests for timber, ranching, or mining. In fact, one of the strongest hopes we have for saving the ancient forests is that their true economic value will now be recognized (McCaleb 1997:236).

In this vein, Cameron (1996) argued that commodifying medicinal plants can be used to improve the economic position of low-status villagers while promoting biodiversity conservation:

> The project will link biodiversity conservation with the marketing of high-altitude medicinal plants in the vicinity of Khaptad National Park in the Seti Zone of far western Nepal....
>
> In light of the rapid destruction of biologically diverse ecosystems and arable land under cultivation throughout Nepal's farming middle hills, improved management of forest ecosystems is urgently needed (Biene et al. 1990; Eckholm 1976). Promoting the sustainable use of ecosystems meets the dual benefits of providing income to local people, as well as conserving and safeguarding the genetic resources housed within them (FAO 1985). It is estimated that, of the over 6,500 species of flowering plants in Nepal, 370 are endemic to Nepal and over 700 species are reported by local people to have medicinal properties (Nepal Environmental Policy and Action Plan 1993:36-37). However, due to the lack of a national program to monitor and protect Nepal's biodiversity, no systematic inventories of the biological diversity of the Khaptad National Park region, (nor of most regions of Nepal in general) exist; thus, it is un-

known how many species of plants and animals are extinct or becoming extinct. Indeed, the establishment of national parks and protected areas, covering nearly eleven percent of the country's total land area, has been Nepal's greatest effort at protecting ecosystems and biodiversity (Cameron 1996:84,85).

While Cameron points out that anthropologists can be effective in facilitating the distribution of profits of commodified plant medicines in ways that are socially beneficial, rather than socially disruptive, she also points out that pharmaceutical corporations are anxious to appropriate local knowledge with little interest in protecting the intellectual property rights of powerless participants or ensuring equitable distribution of any profits that reach local communities.

The pharmaceutical industry and others have indeed capitalized on the conservation movement in order to maximize profit. Yet the merging of the objectives of the pharmaceutical industry with those of environmentalists is commonly represented as being so potentially fruitful, that an alliance which in decades past would have struck many as inherently conflicting, is now viewed by many environmentalists as symbiotic and "natural."

> Among the companies which have embarked on major medicinal plant research programs are Merck, Bristol Myers, Squibb, Pfizer, Monsanto, Smith Klein Beecham, and Eli Lilly. The interest of these companies in as yet undiscovered medicinal plants—or rather, the compounds from medicinal plants—is a testimony to the importance of preserving biodiversity as a source of future medicines.
>
> The most impressive collections of biodiversity are found in true wilderness. Rainforests, whether tropical or temperate, wetlands, and other wilderness areas must be preserved intact to avoid disturbing the delicate balance of these awesomely productive ecosystems (McCaleb 1997:229).

Tied to its objective of profiting through conservation, the pharmaceutical industry has also exploited the scientific research of indigenous plants and medical systems in order to capitalize on indigenous knowledge for Western health needs. For example, ethnobotanists are more likely to get funded to bring back to the Western world medicines which can be commodified in Western markets and medical knowledge that can be developed toward biomedical objectives, or to otherwise provide genetic material to Western scientists. While some attention is given to how tropical plants can be developed into drugs to treat tropical illnesses, this attention remains scant in comparison to how these same plants can be developed into drugs to treat illnesses or unacceptable social behaviors of the industrial world.

This area of research on the part of ethnobotanical science has been criticized for its focus on the commercial potential for Western profit, in which the research itself is value laden but couched as "universal" benefits by way of "discovering" potential cures for disease (Davis 1995). Nonetheless, as Gare (1995:79) points out:

> Through treating things as commodities, the natural conditions for human creativity become private property and are then treated as capital, while people's creative potential is reduced to labor power to be bought and sold on the market.

Nowhere is this more true than in the focus on plant medicines as having monetary value. Such a focus on how plant medicines can be commodified is intended to transform the labor of local communities toward just such ends. Medicines viewed as *economic* resources, exclusive of their social and symbolic resource value, are in this way synonymous with medicines as property, to be bought and sold for profit, and the local medical experts reduced to labor power.

> Increasing American utilization of medicinal plants creates a demand for botanical raw materials which could produce a tremendous boon to farmers, both domestically and abroad....In many cases these botanicals must be produced using ancient and labor intensive methods including hand picking and "garbling," or manual removal of twigs, rocks, and other contaminants from the dried herb. Because of this, these commodities represent a continuing economic opportunity in developing countries for all but the few crops which can be mechanically harvested. According to the U.S. Agency for International Development, the greatest challenge facing most farmers in developing countries is finding markets for crops with sufficient value to sustain a family business. In many parts of the world, agroeconomic development has shifted away from subsistence farming toward the search for specialty crops and cash crops which can be grown on farmland which is currently idle (McCaleb 1997:234).

Thus, the view of forest medicines as inherently good and natural goes hand-in-hand with the global marketing of forest medicines.

The arguments for preserving forest "ecosystems" in order to preserve indigenous medicines and indigenous knowledge may be well intended, but the focus on "indigenous" categories tends to neglect the social differences that characterize every society. Multi-layered social differences at international, state, and local levels determine whose knowledge is accessed and how the benefits of such research and commodification will advantage or disadvantage different members of a society.

By relying on ethnobotanists to legitimate commercial aims as being beneficial to *science* (once issues of intellectual property rights are negotiated and settled, if they are at all), the quest for *scientific* knowledge of the forests' rich pharmacopeia is presented as apolitical and globally beneficial.

> Why should we be so concerned with biological diversity? Consider, for a moment, that knowledge of a relatively small number of species has provided untold benefits to human welfare and the world economy.... Many potential crops and wild relatives of cultivated species remain unknown, and their discovery could have an enormous impact on human welfare and economic productivity (Systematics Agenda 2000: Charting the Biosphere)

While indigenous knowledge of plant medicines does indeed merit respect, attention, and compensation when such knowledge has been appropriated by outsiders, and while botanical research of forest flora and fauna does make a substantial contribution to scientific knowledge and the treatment of many diseases, the scientific process itself is deeply embedded in political concerns.

The political context of science is inherent not only in the questions which are asked—which plants are biomedically efficacious (and therefore can be commodified)—but in which questions are not asked. Why people living in the forest need medicines, why they select plants and not pills, or why they choose pills and not plants, and how the quest for medicine is related to changing ecologies, social structures, and economics, are questions that are not regarded by many policy makers as relevant to understandings of how the forest environment is related to the health of forest residents. Since these questions are considered irrelevant they are generally not asked of forest residents. The end result is that forest residents are expected to depend on indigenous medicines for their health problems as if by "choice" or as "tradition," at the same time they are called on to offer up their medicinal knowledge for gift or sale to outsiders, while receiving no comparable or real access to the pharmaceutical medicines of the industrialized world.

One reason that issues of social structure, economics and politics are not considered by some as germane to the anthropology of medicinal plant use is that the marriage of botany to social science has for the most part focused on how plants are used and valued within the indigenous medical system. Moreover, this focus has relied almost exclusively on either a biological framework (toward understanding the biological value of plant medicines) or on an interpretive framework (toward understanding the symbolic value of plants to those who use them). Davis (1995) summarizes how the merging of ethnobotany and anthropology has evolved:

> Increasingly as ethnologists joined the field, the emphasis shifted from the raw compilation of plant names and uses to an intellectual perspective that viewed the character of a people's relationship with the plant world as but one means of approaching an understanding of the cognitive foundations of a culture.....As anthropologists working in ethnobotany became concerned with the "totality of the place of plants in a culture" (Ford 1978), the intellectual potential of the discipline began to be realized. The study of plants became a vehicle for addressing general issues of ethnological significance. Several themes emerged. The important concept of cultural relativism was reinforced by studies of folk classification, which revealed that aboriginal taxonomies, while not necessarily coinciding with Linnean concepts and categories, were equally complex and firmly rooted in biology (Conklin 1954; Berlin et al. 1974). Studies of hallucinogenic plants offered insights into the origin and character of complex religious beliefs (La Barre 1938; Reichel-Dolmatoff 1971, 1975). Work in medical anthropology highlighted the significance of non-Western concepts of health and healing and, in doing so, emphasized the elaborate connection between spiritual belief, psychological predisposition, and pharmacology that underlies all indigenous practices involving psychotropic preparation (Davis 1995:43).

Thus, ethnobotanical studies provided a much-needed cultural perspective to medicinal plant use which helped Westerners to better understand non-Western cultural practices and beliefs. However, although focusing on the biological and interpretive dimensions of botanical medicines provides critical insights into their local use, such a focus, when it remains isolated from the historical context and the political economy of medicine use, is problematic. Apart from a focus on biological efficacy, by conceptualizing the cultural context of medicines as the cosmological and social *meanings* of medicines, one is almost forced to think in terms of a *shared* concept of reality grounded in a common history and undivided interests. But social categories of class, caste, gender, age and ethnicity shape the social system in such a way that communities are united not just through shared interests and knowledge, but through conflicting ones as well.

Current environmental policies in Madagascar largely ignore social differences and local and national histories in favor of simplistic views that swidden rice production is destroying the forests, it is practiced due to tradition and poverty, and that by educating forest farmers in the practice of irrigated rice production, and increasing their integration into a market economy, they will act rationally which is to say, adopt the new technology and abandon their (irrational) cultural tradition (RNPP 1994; USAID 2001).

Moreover, the World Bank presumes that by investing in human resources, such as health and education, the economic goals of promoting a free market economy in post-colonial nations will be achieved:

> Experience has shown that farmers who have had some primary education achieve higher yields, because they are more receptive to modern methods and are better able to communicate with their suppliers.... Health also has obvious impacts on productivity — healthy farmers can work harder, go further to markets, and so on (World Bank 1994:23).

In short, the linking of health and environment is tied to economic objectives which very much mimic the objectives of colonial states which promoted health and reproductive care in order to ensure a productive labor pool (discussed in Chapter Six). These ideas, that agricultural or health practices are tied to tradition and custom, and can be untied through Western education and introduction to the modern world of technology and chemistry, remain top-down. They do not constitute a form of "cultural exchange" in which education is seen as reciprocal, and indigenous views, behaviors and objectives are regarded as rational, with no need for change by outsiders. Instead, tradition is invoked as an obstacle to modernization.

The fixing of people's beliefs and behaviors as traditional further presumes that they lack the ability to make choices without enlightenment from outsiders (Feeley-Harnik 1991). The desire to reap the rewards of the market economy, however, is presumed to be so universally innate that a project need only facilitate its integration into local economies in order for the culturally-bound native to "choose" to participate.[3]

> Based on the knowledge that the African environment and rural economic growth are inextricably linked USAID programs focus on helping African countries get the conditions right for broad scale investments in practices and systems that increase

---

3. Integration into a market economy was central to the development objectives of many Integrated Conservation and Development Projects (ICDP's), including the Ranomafana National Park Project, and continues to be the foundation on which conservation aid from the United States is based. Further integration into the market economy, and hence, consumption of resources, is regarded as something that will contribute to the conservation of resources.

productivity and reduce environmental degradation (USAID 2001:1)

The principal U.S. interest in Madagascar lies in the high potential of its people to break out of poverty to become one of Africa's emerging market economies, thus enhancing its ability to manage its globally unique biodiversity. Assistance to Madagascar serves U.S. interests by helping establish a legal and policy environment that encourages private initiative and investment, fosters greater respect for human rights and the rule of law, and increases decentralized responsibility for decision making. Assistance to Madagascar also advances U.S. interests by helping the Malagasy people to manage effectively one of the earth's most extraordinary sources of biodiversity.... All of these factors contribute to integrating Madagascar into the world economy and in turn building its capacity to assume a greater partnership role in support of United States interests (USAID January 23, 2001:1).

The potential for economic gain from the rainforest has not been overlooked by those seeking to conserve it. And while human interaction in the ecosystem is viewed by some as "unnatural," it becomes natural when harnessed for commodification. For example, elements within the ecosystem may be viewed as "undiscovered," and their "value" threatened, if they are seen as marketable — either to science, or to consumers. In this view, those living in the "ecosystem" do not "discover" or "value" the rich potential of their forests:

Tropical forests in particular are rich potential sources of valuable foods, medicines, and products of all kinds — if we don't destroy them before their potential can be discovered. When we selectively remove species and damage or destroy entire ecosystems (as in deforestation), resources of enormous potential value are lost... Tropical forests, more than other kinds of ecosystems, remain uncatalogued treasure houses (Erlich and Erlich 1990:101).

As noted earlier, the importance of Madagascar's indigenous plants to international pharmaceutical research and development is well documented. The Malagasy periwinkle, containing a chemical used to treat Hodgins [sic] disease and childhood leukemia, benefits millions of people worldwide. Natural chemical compounds found in many plant species provide vital components for the treatment of disease. Because of the tremendous plant biodiversity found in the remaining rainforests, it is likely that plant species known by western science to be biomedically efficacious, or species which are as yet undiscovered or unexplored by western scientists, exist in the Ranomafana area (RNPP 1994:35).

There are well publicized examples of economic benefits generated through the association of local communities with international pharmacological companies. During the second phase, the natural products development sector of the RNPP will identify potential means of collaboration with both national and international enterprises. While this is an alternative means of increased benefits to peripheral zone communities, three potential constraints will be carefully reviewed; 1) potential non-sustainable harvest of medicinal plants[;] and 2) inequity between local benefits and pharmaceutical profits[;] 3) Malagasy environmental law concerning export/exploitation of beneficial medicinal plants (RNPP 1994:35).

These comments are indicative of many views on the economic and social value of indigenous botanical medicines. Much of the focus on the cultural context of medicines in indigenous communities subjected to conservation or development intervention is made by people trained in the natural sciences or public administration, who often conceptualize culture as something others have, something that is exotic, shared by all members of "the tribe," and fixed in tradition. At best it is agreed that it is important. Indeed, in the best tradition of the missionaries of the nineteenth century, understanding culture is seen by many twentieth century international aid workers—hoping to "improve" economies, environments, and health—as a prerequisite to the success of changing that culture. In the following quote, a nineteenth century missionary suggested that ethnological knowledge of the Malagasy would facilitate enlightenment and economic change:

> There still, however, remains a very marked gap in, at least, our *English* literature treating of the Malagasy ethnology: we know hardly anything definite about those numerous wandering tribes which are popularly known under the name of Sakalava.... Yet these people have many claims upon our attention. They form one of the most numerous of the many different tribes found in Madagascar; they were until the present century the dominant tribe of the country; and they present some strongly marked differences in customs, superstitions, and dialect from those of the inhabitants of the interior and of the eastern coast. It may be hoped that, now [that] we have a Protestant mission established at Mojanga [sic], we shall before long gain some more

accurate information about these Sakalava, who have hitherto been almost entirely untouched by any Christian teaching....

Under enlightened and upright Hova governors, the Sakalava country would recover its prosperity, commerce would be opened up, and the vast agricultural resources of the western provinces would be developed. And last, but not least, Christianity would be introduced, and the people lifted up from their present heathen condition into the light and liberty brought by the Gospel of Christ. We still, however, need much information about the Sakalava tribes (Sibree 1878:456-457,468).

One hundred and sixteen years later, a USAID report reflects little change:

Local customs, traditions and cultural variations can be an obstacle to both conservation and development objectives. The RNPP [Ranomafana National Park Project] will make every effort to identify these forces and work with the recognized community structures to accomplish the objectives that benefit both the communities and the park. Local knowledge will be incorporated into all aspects of the project to heighten the chance of success of activities (RNPP 1994:86).

These quotes suggest that the way the concept of culture has been employed by those seeking to understand other cultures does not necessarily coincide with how this concept is understood by anthropologists. Understanding the distinctive ways in which the term and concept of "culture" has been used by people from varying disciplines and professions may clarify anthropological approaches to the study of culture, health and the environment.

In the following chapter I present an overview of how one experiences the natural and culturally-constructed world of Ranotsara. In this chapter, I show how daily living is fashioned around an environmental landscape that is both breathtaking and life-taking, while those who live within the forest view it as life-sustaining.

Chapter 3

The Research Setting

A Biodiversity of People

The geographical terrain of Madagascar includes tropical, cloud, and montane forests, grasslands, and desert. The island is distinguished by a spine of mountains running longitudinally down its center. The southern regions of the island are dry, barely fertile desert. In other parts of the island, shifting cultivation, primarily of rice, but also of manioc, maize, beans, and other crops, has been practiced with varying intensity since early settlement, combined with pastoral production. Irrigated rice production has also been practiced for many generations, but land suitable for wet-rice production is limited throughout much of the island. Along the coast, fishing supplants agriculture as the primary economic practice.

Although Madagascar is noted for its forest environment, not all Malagasy live in forests. People live in crowded cities, as well as small towns, tiny hamlets, deserts, and coastal fishing villages. The island is peppered with small, seemingly isolated villages that are scattered throughout the mountainous terrain and cut-off by barely navigable rivers or blazing deserts of cactus and sand. Major transportation routes more often resemble a slow-bouncing lunar terrain than the smooth-riding ribbons of concrete Westerners enjoy. The difficulty of traversing the island has led many visitors, both foreign and urban-based Malagasy, to conclude that villagers live lives cut-off from the outside world, a geographical isolation that some believe goes hand in hand with a cultural seclusion. Yet no matter how remote a village, its inhabitants have ridden in cars, listened to radios, maybe even watched television sets. They have all seen well-dressed Asians, Europeans and Americans packing cameras, notebooks, computers, tape recorders, or Bibles. Most rural residents engage in economic exchange of one sort or another with people from other regions, countries, or continents. The concept of "remote" is therefore a bit tricky, as a person can be cut off from roads and communication during certain rainy months of the year, constrained by old age or affliction from going to town for supplies

49

all through the year, and yet at the same time, be economically dependent upon market prices in a town they haven't seen in years or even decades.

Despite the diffusion of villages, towns, and cities, human habitation has been characterized more as an intrusion upon the idyllic Garden of Eden so frequently conjured in images of Madagascar. Harrison (1992:74,75) provides a characteristic summary of how human culture is regarded as a threat to the island's non-human ecology:

> The past serves a clear warning. Within the past two thousand years giant lemurs roamed the mosaic of forest and wooded savannah that once cloaked the plateaux. There were dwarf hippos and a giant tortoise with a shell well over a metre long. And huge elephant birds like the towering *Aepyornis*, chest like a wine barrel, thighs like a horse's, egg big as a football: probable source, through sailor's tales, of the legendary Roc that carried Sinbad off in its talons.
>
> The plateaux are now bare and increasingly barren. The bones are all that remain of the creatures that once lived there. A row of twelve sad skulls in a glass cabinet in Tsimbazaza zoo commemorates the extinct lemurs. The skeletons of *Aepyornis* and dwarf hippo, and the shell of giant tortoise, stand beside them. No major climatic changes occurred that could explain their disappearance. But, some time during the first centuries of our era, longboats sailed over from South East Asia, by way of southern India and East Africa, bringing the first humans to the island.
>
> Within a thousand years of their coming, no land vertebrate heavier than 12 kilogrammes survived. Their habitat, the plateau forest and savannah, was destroyed by fire, turned into pasture for the longhorned, humpbacked Zebu cattle which the settlers brought over, and rice paddies in the valley bottoms. The survivors were hunted to extinction for their meat.
>
> A new wave of extinctions may be imminent. The main threat is the clearance of the rainforests to provide farmland for growing populations.

In all such accounts, whether popular or policy-oriented, the people are not among the island's "wealth," they are not a part of the island's "treasure trove." They are, at best, "friendly," "poor," "uneducated." At worst, they remain fixed in superstition and ignorance, as the following comments of a well-known travel writer attest:[1]

---

1. While travel books are hardly authoritative and are well known to contain distortions, inaccuracies, and a heavy handed dose of romantic imagery, they are important representative texts, particularly in this age of global tourism. Travel books not only encour-

By temperament they are disinclined to look more than twenty-four hours ahead, on any issue (Murphy 1985:151).

While pregnant, Ruth had been advised by her local friends to take extra care as some *ombiasa* [diviners], far out in the bush, still like to get hold of unborn babies; the sun-dried heart and eyes of the unborn are added to their necklaces as particularly powerful charms. This sounds like an extract from one of the more luridly heathen-bashing chapters of the Reverend Matthews or the Reverend Ellis. Yet when I recall the faces of a few of those Mahafaly herdsmen it seemed not entirely impossible that in certain areas such customs survive (Murphy 1985:153).

.... these seemingly easy-going, cheerful, friendly Malagasy are so constrained by a complicated system of beliefs and prohibitions (superstitions, to us) that fear is one of their dominant emotions—even in the 1980s (Murphy 1985:89).

Fortunately casual travelers only need to know that they are dealing with a society far more complex than it looks and to remember that they may be seen as potential dangers because *vazaha* [foreigners] are ignorant of local taboos and could possess mysterious powers to which the Malagasy have no antidotes. This is why so many *fady* [taboos] surround the treatment of *vazaha* and why one's behaviour in a village should, as far as possible, be guided by the people (Murphy 1985:60).

The stereotyping of Malagasy as hopelessly fixed in traditions of ancestor worship, divination, and irrational fear of outsiders, has been used to separate contemporary forest farmers from the recent history and political economy of their regions, including a precolonial autocracy and forced labor, colonial rule, and post-colonial resource appropriation. Just as Murphy could explain Malagasy codes of conduct regarding foreigners as a superstitious fear of their "mysterious" power, with no mention of the history of the three centuries of foreign authority over their land and lives, so too can conservation and development managers explain agricultural practices as "tradition" (RNPP 1994), or one can find in Sierra magazine the following explanation for why the people who live in the forested Ranomafana region do not have enough food:

---

age tourism of foreign lands, but in so doing, they influence the perceptions and actions of tourists who often expect to find superstitious savages, bare breasted or wearing loin cloths. Travel books thus serve to condition the views and interactions of foreign travelers, and they reinforce deeper images of places like Madagascar—places imagined as dark, forbidden and foreboding, untouched by the modern world.

As in much of the tropics, the people living in the Ranomafana rainforest of southeastern Madagascar are the forest's worst enemy, slashing and burning huge swaths of trees to clear land for crops. Plowing the soil would help them raise more food on a single plot of land and let them stop roaming so destructively through the forest, but just teaching people to plow is not the answer here. For the people of Ranomafana, plowing is taboo because it turns the earth's back on God (Knox 1989:81).

The people where I lived howled with laughter when I read them this passage. "We had a plow," 21 year old Lalao explained. "I think it was Faly's [the village leader]. Everyone used it, everyone who could. We liked it, but it only helped a few people with wet-rice fields. You can't use a plow in a *tavy* [swidden] field. I don't know what happened to it. He probably had to sell it, it really wasn't worth keeping, because only a few families could use it. Most people don't have the land for a plow. That is why you don't see one here now; it has nothing to do with Zanahary [God]."

Viewing the economic practices of forest residents as destructive, tied to tradition, and in need of control by outsiders, is not just a view of non-Malagasy. Indeed, urban-based, educated Malagasy are frequently among the most condemning of the practices of their rural compatriots. In the following quote, written by a Malagasy for a WorldWide Fund for Nature (WWF) Report, swidden agriculture is not only viewed as destructive, it is also viewed as a result of the state "giving" forest residents access to the land, an open access regime viewed as innately unmanaged.

Madagascar's enormous biodiversity is extremely important from a scientific point of view. Traditionally our Queen regulated the balance between Man and Nature, deciding on distribution and utilisation of natural resources through a feudal system, whereas the French colonialists laid down clear regulations, but this was no real guarantee of conservation. At independence in 1960 government had strong control of the resources, but in the 1970s people were given free access, which led to severe deforestation and grass burning with resultant soil erosion (Rabetaliana n/d:1).

This quotation illuminates how the forest, and its use, are viewed by the Malagasy state as a national resource to be managed by the state. Conversely, international environmental organizations generally operate under the impression that forests are a "global" resource. By suggesting that species deemed of scientific or economic value must be protected, the 1973 U.S. Endangered Species Act has legislated the rights of U.S. citizens to manage forests outside the boundaries of the United States; this legislation grants Western conservationists the moral authority to intervene in the land management of other countries on behalf of "science" (see Zerner 1996 for a discussion of such conservation narratives). One such effort toward this objective has been unfolding in the southeastern forests of Madagascar, near the village of Ranotsara.

The Ranomafana National Park (RNP) of Madagascar was established in 1990 and managed by the Ranomafana National Park Project (RNPP). As previously indicated, it was administrated largely by U.S. citizens, and financially backed by private and public funding from the United States. Not only is the perception that tropical forests are "global" resources expressed in the rhetoric and discourse of RNP project administrators, the institutional affiliations of the RNPP reflect a view that Madagascar's flora and fauna are of global concern. The RNPP is financially backed by not only USAID, but also by the WorldWide Fund for Nature (WWF), and the MacArthur Foundation, and it is institutionally supported by the World Bank, which funds and monitors the *Association National des Gestations et Areas Protegee* (ANGAP) the national Malagasy institution charged with overseeing national parks and protected areas. While these various institutions deliberate how to best manage Madagascar's forests by volleying reports back and forth between Washington, New York and Antananarivo, the residents of the Ranomafana forest region view the forest in which they live, work and die, as their rightful land to use as they deem fit, a conviction of such force that conservation policies are regarded by forest residents less as policies of protecting the land than as policies of seizing it.

Like many similar conservation and development projects and national parks, and unlike projects and parks which are more participatory in practice, the residents of the Ranomafana forests have been completely excluded from the debates on proprietorship of the land.[2] Moreover, local views of how the forest might be managed have been completely disregarded in favor of preservationist views which regard biodiversity as morally superior to the human lives of the forest ecosystem. These images are difficult for many Americans and others, concerned with the very real and rapid devastation of the earth, to dismiss. Nevertheless, an anthropological study of the ways in which such policies are applied to non-Western cultures may cast light on the social ramifications of prioritizing environmental concerns — as defined by many Westerners — over human ones. Toward this effort, I explore how local, national, and international forces, including policies intended to safeguard the earth's resources and promote

---

2. See Hanson (1997) and W. J. Peters (1997) on how participation has been represented and thwarted by project officials.

economic development, have contributed to the declining health and well-being of many of the world's most disenfranchised people.

The Village and Villagers of Ranotsara

The village of Ranotsara is located in the southeastern montane rain forests of Madagascar, where the altitudinal gradient ranges from 600 to 1200 meters, with an annual precipitation rate of approximately 2900 mm. (Ferraro 1994). While the climate is very hot and dry from about October to the end of December, from January to March, heavy, constant rains begin, including one or more cyclones every year. Such cyclones commonly destroy crops, homes, and even kill people. The threat of cyclones, therefore, is very real to the residents of Ranotsara, who must work daily in the thundering rain, with few clothes for protection, and can still face serious loss should a cyclone destroy their homes or fields. From March through September, the rains continue, gradually becoming much gentler, with intermittent sunny days.

From a distance, Ranotsara is a lovely, quiet hamlet of thatch and tin-roofed homes made of mud, resting amongst banana, coffee, and jack-fruit trees in the center of vast wet-rice fields, often shimmering in the brilliant green of swelling rice. Surrounding these fields rise stony, forested hills, reaching to the celebrated forests of Madagascar, just a ten to twenty minute walk from one's home. The eerie cries of lemurs echo through the village every morning and every evening—the residents readily discern a species just from the sounds it makes as it plays. Children play just as joyfully, and their laughter enlivens the peaceful image of the village, while the rhythmic beating by dozens of women and girls pounding rice, bananas, and coffee provides a steady percussion to mark the time of day.

Reaching the village, a different view envelops the visitor. The people are poor—most wear shredded, filthy rags for clothes; a few wear brightly-colored new clothes imported from the West—Beverly Hills 90210 t-shirts for the boys, frilly acrylic dresses for the girls, one or two digital watches on the wrists of young men. Nearly everyone is at once, both scrawny and strong—while some men are obviously robust and muscular, others are barely heavier than their bones. Yet regardless of the fat on their flesh they are all active—hauling wood, beating rice, planting crops, and carrying children.

Virtually every child has some visible health problem—bellies bloated with worms, noses running, ears oozing white or yellow pus from infection, skin encrusted with scabies lesions, huge boils protruding from legs and arms. Most are coughing or wheezing. A public health survey of the region found that 69 percent of the children under the age of ten were underweight and 11 percent were wasted (having low weight for height) (Kightlinger 1993). The parasite load of children was 97 percent (Kightlinger 1993). Their parents and grandparents are often as sick, and yet they defy the stereotypical image of lethargic, malnourished Africans. Instead, all, young and old, scrawny and robust, hungry and sated, are working, playing, interacting.

The profoundly poor health of the people in an area of such "species rich" forests struck another observer as well. Visiting the newly-established Ranomafana National Park in the early 1990s, environmental writer Paul Harrison noted of Ambodiavy, one of the park's model villages and about ten kilometers from Ranotsara:

> The health of Ambodiaviavy's people is among the worst I have seen in seventeen years of travel throughout the Third World. Half the children were infected with malaria, though only one in six had had fever in the past fortnight. The children delouse one another in lines or circles of four or five. The village is riddled with fleas. It took me three days to get rid of the ones I caught. One in six children has scabies lesions on their hands. One in three has lesions from the jigger flea. The female eats her way into flesh, covers herself with a cyst, and converts herself into a living brood chamber, bloated with her swelling eggs. The hatched larvae eat their way out. Locals pick the cysts out with a pin—but the sore often gets infected.
>
> There are internal parasites. Over 90 per cent of the children have an average of six roundworms, as big as a medium sized garden worm, living in their stomach. One child had a hundred, with a combined weight of 2 kilos. Half have whipworm as well, and a third have hookworm. These parasites consume much of the limited food that the child eats. This contributes heavily to child malnutrition. So does diarrhea—one person in three has an attack in any given fortnight. Almost six out of ten children are malnourished—one in ten severely so.
>
> There are the bleak cases like forty-eight-year-old-Fambelo, who hobbles around on a stick, no longer able to dig his fields, with swollen, aching throat and back pains. He has been seriously ill for a year but hasn't seen a doctor, because he's afraid of the cost in drugs and hospital charges. Blind, landless Miray can afford no treatment or help, but supports his five children working on others' fields, feeling his way (Harrison 1992:86).

Harrison's description of sickness in Ambodiaviavy is not much different than one encounters in Ranotsara, where just as "blind, landless Miray" supports his children by working in the fields of others, foregoing the health treatment he so badly needs, others confront both similar and differing fates and obligations shaping their health in multiple ways.

Living and Working in the Forest

The hard-packed reddish earth of the village landscape is swept or trampled clean each day, while the periphery of the village remains muddied with discarded rice husks and the feces of pigs and children. Chickens and ducks run in and out of homes, pigs are sometimes penned up, sometimes not, sleeping along the edge of a house, passing through the village. Cows periodically pass in herds through the edge of the village, leaving large puddles of feces in the yards of homes, or the paths of residents. Everyone is barefoot—a few in the village own rubber sandals to wear to market on Sundays, but in the village shoes are never worn, and most have never had a pair put on their feet.[3]

There are approximately thirty homes, altogether housing from 180 to about 200 people, a third of them children or teens. Homes are mud-walled and usually thatch-roofed. Some houses have tin roofs, although most of these are rusted and leaking (while a new tin roof reflects cash available to buy it, an older tin roof may or may not speak to wealth; tin was more affordable twenty or thirty years ago, many people could afford it). Most floors are hard-packed earth, some are cement. Woven grass mats are rolled out for company and for sleeping on at night. Often the floors are covered with old worn mats that have settled into the wet dirt floors as if a part of the earth. Most homes measure about five meters by five (though some are as large as nine-by-six), with a wall running through the center to mark off two rooms. Each room has a small window with a wooden shutter to close when it rains. Two of

---

3. While wearing shoes—assuming a resident could even afford them—might cut down on the transmission of parasites, in a village surrounded by rice fields—where it is virtually impossible to get anywhere without wading through rice fields, streams, and rivers—shoes are impractical. Moreover, it remains necessary to remove one's shoes when entering a home—bare feet retain and transmit much less dirt and feces than the soles of a shoe do. To be wearing and removing shoes every time one enters a home, which is to say, several times an hour, becomes tedious, especially since there is no place to leave the shoes during heavy rains—and taking the time to remove them would soak a person even more. While I began my fieldwork adamantly donning the Teva sandals I'd repeatedly been told by many Americans that I ought to wear as if they'd somehow miraculously protect me from parasites, I soon gave them up altogether as I experienced the incredible obstacles they presented in daily village life and going in and out of homes.

the houses are considerably larger, having two stories, with cement floors, vinyl-padded chairs, and even coffee tables. Beds are in most cases a rolled-out grass mat on the earth floor, or laid across a bed of planks in the larger homes. In a few cases, mattresses stuffed with thatch or rice husks (and loaded with bed bugs) provide a soft pallet on which to sleep.

Possessions are few. Grass mats, woven by women every May and June, are the exclusive property of women. So are their pots and pans, although again, these are few, as are their one or two six-quart aluminum covered pots for cooking rice. They may have a smaller four-quart pot for cooking *laoka*, the generic name for any sauce that goes on rice, usually boiled greens or beans, rarely chicken, crayfish, eels, pork or beef. Some baskets, woven yearly like the mats, are used for storing the weeks' or days' supply of rice, coffee, or greens. All women and older girls own a *mpandrary*, a well-worn jaw of a cow, used for smoothing and tightening grass mats. All women have a plastic bucket for hauling water, some have two. Some women have a plastic hair clip, or a pair of earrings, to wear on market day.

Other possessions are the domain of men. They include the dishware, such as a few enamel-covered tin bowls or plates, a few large soup-spoons for eating the rice, maybe a fork or two, two to four tin cups, perhaps one or two plastic glasses for drinking *toaka gasy*, the local moonshine. The men own the large wooden spoons used by women to stir the rice as it cooks, as well as the knife, usually hand-made, also used by women to cut greens or other vegetables. Farming tools are the possessions of men, even though women are as active in farming as are the men. These include spades and knives used for farming and hunting, as well as baskets for catching crayfish, frogs, and eels, empty bottles used for *toaka gasy* or cooking oil, tin lamps to be filled with kerosene, perhaps an old flashlight, usually without batteries. Two homes have radios, which often provide reports of the coming weather or national policies that may affect the farmers. Batteries, when available, are left in the sun (when available), a practice which sometimes helps to charge them. Two homes have hand-powered sewing machines, much prized among the women, although they belong to the men. Men also own the blankets, most families having one or two at most, for the whole family to share. The temperature will often fall to the low forties; cool, wet days are far more frequent than hot and humid ones.

One thing the residents of Ranotsara do not have is garbage. When I first arrived in the village and asked the children where I could throw an empty can, everyone was perplexed. Such a thing would never be thrown away; someone seized it and took it home. Over the next few days I proceeded to collect all my garbage, including plastic wrappers, broken bottles, discarded batteries, wasted note paper, and the like, and asked if there was a place to bury it. Silence was the response, prompting me to ask for a shovel so that I might do it myself. Digging a hole deep into the ground behind my house, I watched in frustration as a crowd encircled me to watch me bury so much old plastic, paper, and broken glass. Never had they had the money to buy so much, much less bury so much. They expressed both disgust that I would be so wasteful (while I was thinking myself ecologically correct for only throwing out what was to me so little), as well as envy that I could be so rich as to throw away so much. It didn't matter — the pigs would root up whatever was buried, and the children turn to toys, or their parents to utensils, all my waste. Eventually, it was rarely necessary to throw anything away, though I continued throughout the year to be the only one with garbage.

Other prized possessions include any type of cannister that can be tightly closed. Because rice and soap are two of the favorite meals of rats, having a means of securing them is a genuine need. Nestlé milk tins, rare due to the egregious cost of the product, are among the most prized, while any type of cannister discarded by foreigners will do the trick. But having tightly-closed cannisters or containers big enough to store rice, or small enough for soap, was rare. Often women would find that the soap or medicine they'd purchased (at a price which they couldn't afford) had been eaten at night by the rats. Rice was often eaten as well, although bananas could be hung out of reach. One woman brought her baby boy to me to show me how a rat had nibbled his foot in the night and he hadn't even woken. Another woman, Soa, showed me the scars on her foot left by a rat that had bitten her in her sleep. She giggled as she described it. "I felt it, but I was too tired to do anything but kick it," she explained. I told her I thought it was horrible to be bitten by a rat in your sleep. "That's true," she conceded, "but that is our life, I was happy it ate me and not the rice." She giggled again and asked me if I had any *toaka gasy* to drink.

Children's possessions include two different types of sling-shots. The wooden and rubber-laced Y-shaped sling-shot is owned by boys. The other type is a macraméd cord which girls use. Both types of slingshots are used to shoot at birds which infest the rice fields, or to catch birds or small animals for eating.

Toky was twelve years old, but looked about nine; with a grin the size of a crescent moon, and a belly like a watermelon he was so bloated with worms. Toky is a survivor. His father had died when he was six, and he learned at an early age to take over the tasks of the household while his mother worked in the fields. He chopped and hauled wood for cooking, made his own breakfast, lunch, and dinner of boiled green bananas, of which he never tired. He roasted his own rice for snacks and cared for his little brother, iPauly, throughout the day. There really isn't much that Toky cannot do—he is clever, ambitious, and the best story teller in the village.

But he is very poor, and not having the money to buy a length of rubber, which cost about ten cents, he had no sling shot. When I learned that several of the boys in the village were in the same spot as Toky, not having what was one of the most basic tools of a young boy's daily living, I invested about two bucks and bought them all rubber.

Toky was probably the proudest boy in the village with his new sling-shot, which he made from the limb of a tree after I gave him the rubber. He proved such a fine craftsman at it, that he soon found himself teaching the other boys how to make their own. Once done, Toky boasted daily of the birds he'd caught in the rice fields, or the small animals he'd shot to feed his family. "But don't worry," Toky told me, "I won't use it on Masobe," he said with a grin, referring to my neighbor who was forever snitching coffee, sugar, or oil from me. And then the grin vanished and a most serious look came across his face, "unless..." and Toky's giant eyes slowly sailed toward Masobe's house, the threat dangling in the air for just a moment too long, before he picked up the sling-shot, mimed a shot at Masobe, and rolled on the floor cackling.

One day, a French tourist who had been hiking through the hills arrived out of the blue. He was given a place to sleep in an unused room of a cement-floored home. He kept to himself and showed little interest in the residents. Toky, who had been learning English from me, was most eager to show off his new but limited language skills, not quite understanding that white people often come from different parts of the world. As far as Toky was concerned, this was another *vazaha* (foreigner), he was white, he spoke a funny language, he must be like me. Besides, I could speak to him (in French), so why couldn't Toky speak to him as well (in English)? What I had failed to explain to Toky was that French and English are two different languages, and that this man did not speak English.

Toky went to visit him, taking his new sling-shot to show off. He came back shortly, very unhappy.

"*Sady-be ianao* [you are very sad]," I said to him, "*inona ity* [what is it]?" I asked.

Toky explained that he had gone to the *vazaha's* room and tried to talk to him, but the man had no interest in talking to him, he was more interested in reading his book filled with pictures of lemurs and birds.

"*Maka* sling-shot!" he said, telling me he was going to take his sling-shot, his favorite new word in English, and continuing in Malagasy, "shoot the tourist, because he is not a real *vazaha*."

"How do you know he is not a real *vazaha*?," I asked him.

"Because he does not even know the word *sling-shot*," he said, emphasizing again the English word. "I will tell the police he is a spy, or comes from another world. *Everyone* knows *sling-shot*," he exclaimed, shaking his head in amazement at the tourist's ignorance of this most basic word. A sling-shot was, to Toky, the most basic of human possessions, and to not recognize one was practically unhuman. And with that, Toky, more gentle and rare than a Golden Bamboo Lemur, launched into a comical pantomime of doing away with the tourist with his sling shot (right through his eye ball), chopping up his body with a kitchen knife, washing the knife clean, chopping down and hollowing out a tree in which to hide his body, and finally tossing the tree—loaded down with imaginary rocks—into the Namorona river.

Suddenly, a sputtering of incomprehensible babble sprang from Toky whose eyes flared with rage as he jumped up with his sling shot and shook it fiercely. And just as suddenly Toky's face changed to one of innocence and fear, as he threw himself on the floor and looked up to an invisible presence, imploring with his sling shot held between his folded hands, "*fa tsy olona izy* [but he was not human]," he cried, "*tsy fantany* sling-shot! [he did not know sling shot!]" he explained, and with that Toky rolled again on the floor laughing hysterically.

(He repeated this story, with more and more elaborate variations on the concealing of the body and the interrogation by the police, for several evenings afterwards. It took me the longest time to figure out what the incomprehensible babblings were—his version of a policeman speaking English, a disturbing reminder that authority, in Toky's world, speaks in a foreign tongue).

While the sling shot is perhaps the most basic possession of both boys and girls, other possessions of children include their school books, a pen or pencil, a notebook for their homework, and sometimes homemade wooden toys. One of the most common such toys are hand-crafted wooden blocks which the children called "cassette radio," and which they carried with them, pushing wooden "buttons" and singing their own songs.

The only other possessions the people of Ranotsara might have would be tools of the trade, such as plates, coins, or mirrors, used by *ombiasa* (shamans) for divining misfortune or sickness, a globe owned by one of the teachers, or cow horns owned by *mpanjaka* (village leaders) and used for offering ceremonial *toaka*. A few young men owned *kabosy*, hand-crafted wooden ukeleles, which were often brought out for planned or spontaneous parties.

Perhaps the most prized possession of both men and women are *lamba*, or brightly-colored cloths. *Lamba* are used for clothing—wrapped over clothes, or worn alone as skirts or dresses for women. They are also used for carrying children on the back, tied like a sling. And most importantly, *lamba* are used to wrap the dead. When Soa's husband, Lita, died from what appeared to be hepatitis, I remarked on how few clothes he and his family had during his life, yet now that he was dead he had many *lamba*. Lalao, a young woman and friend replied, "Yes, that is the Malagasy *fomba* [custom]. You have no *lamba* when you are alive and need clothing, but when you are dead and need nothing, you will be well-dressed!" She appreciated the irony of having nothing until death, yet having nothing to be buried in would be an even crueler fate.

Clothing is limited for everyone. Some have a good set of clothes, for going to market or wearing at ceremonies, but not everyone. Yet most people have at least a change of clothes, to wear when the others are washed.

Tsaralahy was one of the people who had no change of clothes. Six years old, skinny as a stick, Tsaralahy had a raggy pair of shorts to wear, without so much as a button or piece of elastic to hold them up. He could always be seen clutching his little shorts as he ran, trying to hold them up while he played ball, stood in the doorway, walked to school. Although I employed his mother, and gave her cloth and buttons, Tsaralahy's shorts were never repaired or replaced. In fact, they eventually disappeared altogether, and Tsaralahy, covered with scabies lesions within a few months, was naked twenty-four hours a day.

"Why doesn't his mother use the *lamba* [cloth] I gave her to make him some new shorts?" I asked some of the women.

"*Tsy fantatro* [I don't know]," one answered. "She likes the cloth for herself. She drinks *toaka* [homemade rum]."

I remained puzzled about Tsaralahy and why he had no clothes. I asked repeatedly why his mother did not make him clothes. She always assured me she would. I asked repeatedly why others did not intervene. But no one could or would give me a clear answer. The school teachers had done their best, one of them, Bodo, explained. "We told her that he was ashamed to come to school because he has no clothes. We told her that he would need clothes to attend school."

"What happened?" I asked.

"He stopped coming to school."

Tsaralahy's mother finally relinquished the *lamba* she had been wearing, which I had given to her to make her son's shorts, when she wrapped Tsaralahy for burial on New Years Day. Like so many other children in the village, including those well fed and well-clothed, malaria hit suddenly and hard, and left his parents wounded and deeply scarred. Yet the story of Tsaralahy is baffling because a child is so loved in Madagascar, that to neglect one is both rare and incomprehensible. As I show in Chapter Eight, however, Tsaralahy's neglect, and the community's failure to intervene, were not the only such incidents I witnessed. One question I cannot answer remains, did his mother so prize *lamba* that she would reserve it for herself, rather than convert it to shorts for her son?

The answer matters little, as the *lamba* could not have saved Tsaralahy, but the medicine his parents desperately sought as his life gave way may well have.

Daily Activities

Just as dying is done in the home, so too is cooking, on a three-stoned fire pit over which corn, tobacco or, rarely, strips of beef or eel, hang to smoke. In some cases, there are separate homes for cooking, and in a few cases, cooking is done outside, under an open-walled thatch roof. The walls and ceilings of homes in which one cooks are a lacquered-black from the smoke, with soot-covered cobwebs enshrouding the rafters. As light penetrates the small square of window, the sunlight illuminates the cobwebs with an intriguing soft beauty, as if the home were draped from corner-to-corner with filaments of silk. The dried ears of corn suspended over the fire glow with shining black and golden kernels. The smoke from the fire drifts and curls into the sun, while an infant sitting by his sister may pee a barely noticed trickle of urine onto the floor, an older man might spit in a corner, a rat might pass unhurried along a wall. A tin cup is wiped clean with an old rag and dipped in a pot of coffee, sweetened with sugar the hosts cannot afford, and offered to the guest.

Concepts of health and cleanliness are different here, where a bar of soap costs a day's wages, water doesn't run from the tap, and there is hardly any dry land twenty meters from a house on which to build a latrine. The homes rest on an island amongst the rice fields, and a grove of coffee trees provides the village with a natural and somewhat private "latrine," with special areas for children and sick people.

Moreover, keeping clean is a continual challenge for farmers, who labor in wet-rice fields, where the mud is calf-deep, and thick with worms and feces, or they work in the hillsides, digging, planting, and chopping in the blazing sun. Women pound rice, bananas and coffee up to two hours a day before it is even ready to cook. Children learn to crawl and walk in the mud and dirt, because they have no alternative. Babies have no diapers—cloth is too expensive, and so is the soap to wash them.

Keeping clean is a challenge. Still, as with everything, people differ in the importance they give to cleanliness. To be clean may be having hair that does not smell bad, or to have bathed within the last few days. Living as forest farmers, one could be covered with mud and still be clean, if one's body had been washed recently, just as one could be mud and dust free, but still be considered dirty, if one had not had a bath and smelled foul.

Even given this definition of cleanliness, some people are cleaner than others. In general, older people placed more importance on bathing and cleanliness than did younger people. This was variously attributed to the indifference of youth, the stress that the colonialists and missionaries placed upon cleanliness in the past, and the growing poverty that makes keeping clean when one's workload increases, and yet has less money for soap, such a constant challenge that it is easier to give up and live with filth, than to combat it.

While I heard no end to the explanation for poor hygiene, sickness, and even poverty, as being due to the people being *kamo*, or lazy, this explanation (usually offered by Malagasy elite or Americans) was hardly plausible, given the daily lives of the residents. The local economy is based on farming and as such, everyone works from sunrise to sundown in the management of their environments. Women rise at about four-thirty or five, nurse their babies, go to the river to bathe and bring back water for cooking. Older girls (from the age of about eight) pound the rice for breakfast, as their mothers start the fire (their husbands or sons having chopped and brought firewood), boil the water, clean the newly pounded rice, cook it, and prepare some greens if they are available. More often, breakfast is boiled green bananas or manioc, because for all the rice that is grown it is not enough for three meals a day all through the year. The entire region has been a net importer of rice since the mid-1980s (Ferraro 1994), a period coinciding with the advent of structural adjustment policies (discussed in more detail in Chapter Four).

After the breakfast dishes have been taken to the river and washed, children go to school, while their parents begin working the rice fields; older women will usually remain at home to watch over the young children, sort beans, and cook, while older men (and sometimes women) may just gossip and drink *toaka*, or they may participate in housing repair and construction. Growing poverty and social change has recently forced some older people to work in the rice fields of the wealthier residents, for wages of approximately 30 cents a day. For the most part, everyone is active and most engaged in hard labor, and this hard labor is centered around agricultural production of rice.

How the production of rice has been represented by various writers and policy makers, however, is in sharp contrast to the way that it is experienced by those who work the fields. Inextricably linking swidden rice farming to the changing forest cover in Madagascar, the standard representations of *tavy* are those of destruction.

The Forest and the Land

The term for swidden agriculture in Madagascar is *tavy*, and, ignoring the history of rapid industrialization, mining, and export production in nineteenth century Madagascar (discussed in detail in Chapter Four), it is a term conjured continuously to "explain" deforestation in Madagascar. *Tavy* is typically described as follows:

> With 90 percent of the forest gone, uncounted species have lost their habitats and become extinct, and most of the soil cover has been lost to erosion.
>
> This destruction is largely due to slash-and-burn agriculture. People are constantly burning the rain forests for agricultural purposes—it is the way they make a living. First, the villagers burn the virgin rain forest and plant crops in the fertile burned areas. But since the soil loses its fertility in 3 or 4 years under these conditions, fields soon cease to be productive and so the farmers move on to another patch of rain forest and begin the cycle again (Wright 1993:451).

Most images of *tavy* that are presented to the public focus on its destructive aspect—and it is, indeed, destructive to forest cover. Photos of *tavy* suggest burned hillsides, trees reduced to stubble. References in policy documents, and academic and popular articles, refer to it as "slash-and-burn," illuminating the practice of chopping the trees, burning the "virgin" forest, and "abandoning" the burnt fields. This image, however, does not correspond to the image of *tavy* that many farmers hold. Farmers refer to *tavy* as inter-cropped fields, yielding rice, manioc, maize, beans, greens, and other crops. Indeed, as I walked along a dirt path with twelve-year old Soary, she pointed to a field of ripe manioc, and asked me to take a photo, telling me that *tavy* is not just burned earth, which we had just passed and I had photographed, it is also food and therefore, life.

The life of the forest, then, is inseparable from the lives of the residents. While the forest is typically characterized as an intact ecosystem threatened by encroaching *tavy* farmers, it is viewed differently by the people who live and work within in. To the residents of Ranotsara, the *ala*, or forest, is the land on which their ancestors lived and died, and their current source of sustenance. Viewing the forest as both their past, present, and future, they do not see themselves as outside it—rather, they view those who seek to keep them out of it as outsiders of the forest.

In addition, the forest is not perceived by the residents of Ranotsara as a bounded environment—the forest extends to the village, having multiple terrains, textures, and transitions. What I and others have termed "the village" is to the residents the *tanana*, or community (itself a problematic concept, with ever-changing patterns of residence and alliance that I discuss in more detail in Chapter Six).

The *tanana* is a part of, or within, the forest landscape. Dense forest, incorrectly termed "virgin" forest by many Westerners seeking to capture a paradoxical image of undefiled growth, is more precisely termed *ala be* [great forest] by those who live with the trees. As the forest is transformed from a landscape of undomesticated to domesticated sustenance through the process of *tavy*, it passes through stages. Whereas an etic view of swidden horticulture speaks of plots left fallow, the Malagasy forest farmers view regenerating land as *jinja*; as this land is planted with cash crops, it becomes *hibohibo*. Each of these stages is valued for providing essential resources to those who manage the "fallow."

Tavy itself has two stages, as Hanson (1997:36) explains:

> *Mitavy ala* and *mitavy kapoka* are the two phrases used to describe the clearing, burning and planting of primary forest and healthy secondary forest respectively. The Tanala also refer to swidden as *manazava tany* (to make the land clear) and *manadio tany* (to clean the land). The ambivalent and complex attitudes the Tanala maintain toward forested land is apparent as one considers these phrases. For while forested land is thought to be "cluttered" and "wild", vegetation is also the sign of land that is still fertile — land that still has *tsiro* (taste).

Tavy, therefore, is as much a part of the forest environment and process as is a dark and tangled grove of trees. The forest is alive and moving, and differing faces of the forest provide differing needs.

The contrast between local views of the land and forest, and state and project views of the forest as a degraded landscape caused by swidden farming, is not limited to Madagascar. Fairhead and Leach (1996) noted that scientists and policy-makers have, since the late nineteenth century, considered the patchy landscape of Guinea's forest cover to reflect a process of continued degradation, also associated with swidden farming. Incorporating historic photographs of the region with maps and local narratives, the authors found that contrary to representing a progressive loss of forest cover, the patchy landscape was, in fact, a reflection of both stable and progressive forest growth. That is, despite the received view that there had been an original vegetative state from which the present landscape could be used to infer degradation, forest cover had either been relatively stable or had actually increased with time. Fundamental to the received view, they suggest, is the fallacy of a climatic climax vegetation in which there exists a state of "natural" vegetation in a given region, which remains unchanged except by human interaction.

Fairhead and Leach (1996) argue that contemporary environmental policies reflect prejudices and assumptions of colonial science, in which local inhabitants were assumed to be ignorant of the land, and colonial administrative policies regarding land and resource control shaped ways of thinking about local land and resource practices. The objectives of colonial policy thereby influenced the methodologies of colonial science, leading to "scientific" legitimation of uninformed assumptions.

> Colonial science developed not only ideas concerning forest loss, but also methodologies for elucidating vegetation change which became and have remained 'authoritative'. Central has been the deduction of long-term change from snapshot or short-term observations, inferring process from form. Thus it is that forest islands appear as relics indicating a historical process of forest loss; a deduction now made not only from on-the-ground botanical, forestry and vegetation survey observations, but also when forest islands appear in remotely-sensed imagery (Fairhead and Leach 1996:114).

Fairhead and Leach point to the need for historical research to understand the different processes that shape how landscapes change unevenly. Feeley-Harnik (1995:55fn) raises this same point for Madagascar, suggesting that remote-sensing analyses of the island have been used to attribute changes in forest cover in the eastern regions of Madagascar, without addressing problems related to the baseline data such analyses use to assess rates of deforestation. She points to how reports of deforestation trends in Madagascar regard Malagasy agriculturalists as an undifferentiated group, and have not considered the major historical transformations of land use and land tenure in Madagascar, processes which have contributed to the complexity of present land use practices.

Feeley-Harnik suggests that the faulty methodology of science has been incorporated into contemporary conservation policy in Madagascar. In this same way, Fairhead and Leach (1996) find that in West Africa, the popularity of conservation movements have enabled the contemporary Guinee state to continue replicating colonial science.

> Scientists and others have also repeatedly observed Kissidougou's landscape from a social position which made forest destruction logical, and attention to local inhabitants' opinions difficult or unimportant. Racialist, pejorative views of African farming and forestry practices came to dominate Guinee's colonial administrations. The preconceived opinions and hurried visits of today's foreign experts, and the attitudes and training of urban-based state functionairies, compound such views. It can be argued that the image of the rural farmer as environmental destroyer, and hence the need for modernization of resource management and farming techniques, conforms to and

helps to justify the self-distinction of urban intellectuals as 'modern' and progressive; distinctions reinforced under the First Republic when the urbanized were politically and economically privileged, and their vision of a highly mechanized, capital-intensive technical future dominated approaches to rural development [Riviere, 1971] (Fairhead and Leach 1996:114, 115).

Feeley-Harnik (1995:45) echoes this comment, "Yet the older arguments opposing plants to people, and primordial 'slash-and-burn' planters to modern world citizens, persist."

Land management practices in rural areas are indeed much more complex than representatives of the state or conservation projects may represent them to be. In the case of Madagascar, the process of *tavy* cultivation is not the simple, lazy-man's habit of growing a garden that the term "slash-and-burn" suggests, but is instead a labor-intensive agricultural strategy that regenerates the land as much as depletes it.

The Agricultural System of the Ranomafana Region

Hanson (1997:37-39) provides a model description of how farmers manage the *tavy* process—and how this labor contrasts with how it is perceived by outsiders. His description merits quoting at length:

Contrary to the implications of the phrase 'slash-and-burn', *tavy* land preparation proved to be a complex process indeed. In late August, Botovelona began chopping down the small trees and larger shrubs constituting the forest under story (*manaratsaka*, or *tavy zanakazo*). Then, working with a large ax (*famaky, andronana*), he felled the larger trees (*mandavo sangy*), careful to direct them in such a sway that they might help prevent soil erosion during the torrential rains. For a month and a half, Botovelona waited for the newly cut vegetation to dry in the sun (*manaina tavy*), and in mid-October, he burned (*manoro tavy*). Before burning, Botovelona prayed to Zanahary [God] and the forest spirits (*fahasivy*) to request permission to burn. After waiting for a few days for the land to "cool", Botovelona then went through the field checking for trees that were not dried in the fire.

In November, Botovelona, his immediate family, and those relatives he could enlist from his kin cooperative began planting. Before planting, however, Botovelona performs a *sao-tany sotra* (a simple thanks to the earth), asking Zanahary and the forest spirits for their blessing. Then the planters move in a line across the steep field poking a stick sharpened at one end (*fitomboka*) into the ground and dropping two to three seeds into the holes. In the first *tavy* planting, Botovelona plants rice, preferably *toamasina* or *tomborongo*—the two preferred varieties of upland seed. *Beingizina* and *vary malady* are also planted in the *tavy*, yet these are generally less favored. The first rice is often intercropped with cucumber, corn, and various greens. In January and February, the fields must be weeded (*miava*). The guarding of the field against *fody* [birds] occurs in March and April, and the field is finally harvested in April and May. The reaping of *tavy* rice is variously labeled *mipitika vary*, *misongo vary*, and *mila vary* and involves clipping the tops of the plants (the *salohim-bary*) with a small knife (*karima*). *Tavy* rice yields in the first year are generally low, averaging 0.5tons/hectare (RNPP 1990:6). Botovelona now waits until August to once again weed the field and to turn it over into clods (*manifikifika*). He waits two weeks and burns the plot again. In September, Botovelona plants beans and corn and harvests these crops in December. After planting rice in his *tavy* field for two years in a row, Botovelona faces a number of choices. He can go ahead and plant rice for another 2-3 years, intercropping it with a wide range of vegetables. However, this choice quickly deteriorates the soil's fertility. He may decide, on the other hand, to dedicate the plot to bananas or coffee trees. While bananas generally take only one year to produce results, coffee can take up to seven or eight. If Botovelona does choose the cash crop option for his field, he can no longer plant rice there and must look for an additional plot. The decision faced by the farmer after two years of rice in a *tavy* field is influenced by such factors as whether or not he has other plots to work with and if he can readily borrow rice during the period his cash trees grow.

The complexity of the options facing Botovelona in his *tavy* field stand in stark contrast to most representations of *tavy* farming in Madagascar as easy and simple. Nothing could be further from the truth. In fact, the farmer's strategy of how, when, and what to plant in his upland fields could spell the difference between famine and survival should a heavy storm during the cyclone season submerge and rot his valley crops.

"Deforestation" and even "the forest," then, are complex concepts, which project administrators have made little effort to understand. Hanson's perspective reveals a sharp contrast from those who have already defined the problem.

My own conversations with residents similarly revealed that contrary to not understanding the processes of environmental degradation associated with swidden production, the residents of Ranotsara are more concerned with forest land than forest trees, because it is the land that sustains them. "We need the land," Masobe, an elder village male explains, "but not the forest. But the land is not enough, if we do not have enough workers to work the land." Masobe understands the value of workers—his wife has died, and his only living child residing in the village has, like many others, begun working for wages of 1,500 fmg a day (about 30 cents at the time of my research), for a wealthier resident who owns irrigated rice fields.

Bodo, a 32 year old village school teacher and mother of five girls, elaborates. "Land is more important than the trees. Even though we have learned about the animals in the forest, we need food more than trees. There are people who don't have *tanim-bary* (irrigated rice fields) and so they need *tavy*. And for those who have *tanim-bary*, they need chemical inputs. For those who are poor, who don't have *tanim-bary* or the money for chemical inputs, they need the forest for *tavy*."

Masobe and Bodo's suggestions that the land and trees are separate does not mean that they do not understand the ecological relationship between land and trees. As Hanson's description reveals, *tavy* farmers possess sophisticated understandings of the interrelationship between land and trees and that trees are necessary to prevent erosion. But they have been presented with a conservation ethic that itself separates trees from land, by emphasizing the value of trees over that of the soil on which the trees grow. In response, Masobe and Bodo have sided with the soil, and their rights to determine what grows from it.

When sufficient land is available to farmers for allowing *tavy* fields to remain fallow for ten to fifteen years (which some outsiders refer to as "abandoning"), it proves to be a sustainable agricultural strategy. Nonetheless, as populations have been forced to settle in villages and remain stationary, and as current privatization of lands have prevented farmers from migrating, the land base has been diminished, fallow periods shortened, and more and more people forced to increase *tavy* production.

The current agricultural system employed by subsistence farmers combines *tavy* with irrigated rice agriculture and cash crop production. Rather than representing three different types of agricultural systems, the land is farmed as a single system in which three different cropping strategies are practiced simultaneously to maximize yields. In Ranotsara, the majority of farmers where I lived owned *tavy* fields exclusively, lacking the labor and suitable land for irrigated rice, while a minority owned (or rented) irrigated rice fields. Most all had some sort of cash crop land, such as bananas or coffee.

The daily work is seasonal, yet certain patterns are maintained. The wet-rice fields will be prepared by the men using *angady*, long-handled, narrow-based spades, after cattle have trampled the fields (while a generation ago every family owned cattle, now only three families in the village have any cows, with most belonging to one family, to be discussed subsequently). *Tavy* fields are cleared with *antsy-be* (big knives), and burned, after which tree roots are dug up by men.

After the fields are prepared for sowing, women and young girls work in teams to plant the rice. This can be very arduous work, because it requires being bent over for hours at a time. Moreover, the wet-rice fields are infested with parasites and feces, making it an unhealthy environment in which to work. Once the rice has been planted, it must be weeded daily. While weeding is primarily the responsibility of women, the recent shift to wage labor in Ranotsara has necessitated some men and young boys to begin participating in this activity, as well as older women who would have, in prior years, retired from heavy labor in favor of domestic responsibilities.

When the crops are mature, they must be harvested, which is the responsibility of both men and women. *Tavy* rice is the easiest to care for and to harvest, although the steep terrain of the fields make it a bit difficult to work. *Tavy* rice is cut off in stalks with a small home-crafted blade, while a large sickle is used for cutting wet-rice. While both men and women will cut *tavy* rice, only men and boys cut wet-rice. Women and girls then thresh the rice to remove it from the stalks. The rice is then ready to dry in the sun, later to be stored and pounded.

Other crops that must be planted, weeded, and harvested include beans and manioc, both important dietary staples. In addition, most families either own, or tend, banana and coffee trees, which provide an important cash crop.

The farming activities of all adult men and women can take from four to eight hours of every day; the only time they have off is in the event of a death (in which case all but essential work ceases for three days), if there is an important festival, or if a governmental representative or healthcare worker comes to the village. In addition to the daily farming and cooking activities, water must be hauled from the river at least twice a day, clothes must be washed, children cared for, houses repaired, medicines collected and prepared, firewood collected and chopped, fish traps set in the river, tools crafted, and trips made to the market to purchase supplies or sell crops. The day usually ends at sundown for the men, a bit later for the women who must wash the dinner dishes.

The Labor and Education of Children

It is not possible, however, for the adults of the village to finish a day's work in a day. The labor of children is vital to the productivity of the household and village. Children contribute to the household by watching younger children (primarily the responsibility of girls, but also of boys), by helping prepare the meals (in some cases, preparing them alone, while their parents work the fields), pounding the rice, collecting and chopping wood, and working in the fields for wages and meals, or if their parents are fortunate enough to own and control their own fields, by assisting their parents.

About one-quarter mile from the village is the two-room village school. Two resident teachers instruct two levels of students; lessons include reading, writing, and mathematics. There is minimal instruction beyond that. Few children or youths can recognize Madagascar on a world map, while I found none who were locally educated who could identify Africa, the United States, or France. Nonetheless, school is vitally important to most every parent, who will sacrifice her or his own needs in order to pay for a child's pencils and notebooks. In addition, the school teachers have few supplies of their own, and must depend upon very old curriculum guides, limited chalk, and tattered foam for erasers.

School begins after breakfast, and lasts until about three, with a two hour break for lunch. After school, most children take their sling-shots to the rice fields and scare off the birds as they feed at the end of the day. Other children go to the forest to catch insects or small game for protein, while others (young boys) go to the forest to tend the cattle and guide them from field to field.

Regional Links

Administratively speaking, Ranotsara is situated in the *faritany* (province) of Fianarantsoa, with the *fivondronana* (sub-province, or local political seat) in Ifananadiana, approximately 32 kilometers east of Ranotsara. Despite its proximity, Ifanadiana remains distant. The nearest road is Highway 25, which runs 205 kilometers from Fianarantsoa in the southern highlands, to Mananjary on the eastern coast. Highway 25 is about a one-and-a-half hour strenuous hike from Ranotsara. To reach Ifanadiana, one must first hike the eight kilometers over the mountains to the main road, await a local *taxi-brousse*, pay 6,000 fmg for one-way fare (approximately $1.50 at the time of my fieldwork, and representing four to five days' wages for most villagers), and hope that business can be taken care of in time to catch a *taxi-brousse* returning, for which one must pay an additional 6,000 fmg.

Such a trip often requires spending the night with extended family or friends in Ifanadiana, in order to take care of all business and get back before nightfall, then hike the hour-and-a-half over the mountains to return to the village. In the rainy season, such a trip is often very difficult, if not impossible. In addition to having to hike and climb over the slippery muddied path, there are three rivers to be crossed; in the rainy season, one of these rivers must be crossed by way of a long single log set across the banks of the river — requiring a challenging balancing act on the slick wet trunk, particularly difficult if one is carrying a child on the back, a basket of bananas on the head (to be sold at market), and a toddler in the arms. This river alone discourages many women from even making the trip, regardless of its necessity (while others skip merrily along defying gravity).

A second river is crossed by wading knee-to-waist deep across its width, but then one reaches the massive Namorona river, which must be crossed by way of a bamboo raft, similar in design to a *pirogue*. Not everyone, however, knows how to maneuver the raft, particularly women. Consequently, when one reaches the river, if the raft is waiting and they or someone accompanying them knows how to steer it, they can cross without problem. On the other hand, if the raft is on the other side of the river, with no skipper in sight, or if the raft is available but a skipper is not, then one must wait. Because the path from the villages to the main road is heavily traveled, such a wait is never very long, no more than an hour at most, (unless the sun is setting, in which case, travelers have returned home, except for the occasional drunken youth or late-comer).

During the rainy season, however, this raft is frequently unavailable. The heavy torrential rains that pour from January to April (continuing, though much lighter, until October), as well as frequent cyclones, often destroy the raft. During my stay it was not uncommon for the raft to be repaired one morning, only to be destroyed the same night. A communal effort contributes to the maintenance of this raft. Young men from the five villages that depend upon it take turns repairing it or building a new one; unfortunately, every time it came the turn of the men from Ranotsara to repair the raft, it remained unavailable for weeks at a time. Residents from other villages continually chided the men from Ranotsara for their laziness, a reputation that was even invoked by project representatives to explain the alarming death rate. The men from Ranotsara responded that it was useless to repair the raft, it would only be smashed the following night, so why bother? Instead, they could wade shoulder-deep across the river, as long as they followed the safest route, or they could hike through the cane fields to the shallowest spot in the river, having no need of the raft.

The route through the cane fields, however, is very narrow, difficult, and almost impossible to traverse for pregnant women or women with small children. Moreover, it is a favorite haven of boa constrictors, which most women fear (there are no poisonous snakes in Madagascar, but they do get to be very big). As such, when the raft was gone and it was up to the men of Ranotsara to repair it, you could be sure that it would be a while and the women would be angry. Sometimes, residents of one of the other villages would get tired of waiting and they would go ahead and repair it, other times, it might be a month before a raft was repaired. At any rate, the raft to cross the river was a continuous obstacle to travel, and during the rainy season a trip was never ventured without inquiring as to whether or not there was a raft.

Despite the difficulties one encounters in order to reach the main highway, trips to Ifanadiana are essential for the two local schoolteachers, at least one of whom must go there every month to collect their governmental pay — often to find no one available to distribute the money, and therefore requiring an overnight stay until someone shows up who can pay them. And anyone wishing to register land, as the national policy of land privatization requires, must go there. Anyone wishing to access dental services must go there. Anyone needing any health care beyond the most basic primary care must go there, or at least to Ranomafana. Anyone needing to press civil or criminal charges against someone, or having such charges pressed against them, must go there. In short, trips to Ifanadiana are frequently necessary, and entail considerable time, effort, and money.

The nearest and most commonly-used market for residents of Ranotsara lies also along the main road, just across the Namorona river. For most farmers of Ranotsara, the hamlet of Moratoky is where rice, bananas and coffee will be sold, and oil, soap, sugar, or petrol purchased. The town of Ranomafana is about a ten-minute walk from Moratoky, and situated along the main road. Its role as a market center has taken a back seat, however, to the town's role in international conservation. It now serves as the local administrative center for the Ranomafana National Park. Hence, those who cross the forested hills to sell their bananas or their coffee, to purchase some cooking oil or petrol for a tiny flame by which to see their children's faces in the night, have in recent years seen foreigners from every continent, some with cameras around their necks, others with lap top computers and cocktails on the veranda, still others leaping in and out of Toyota land cruisers to catch a quick lunch of crawfish and rice on their way to paradise and back again by the time the sun goes down, the report of their encounters in the wild written and submitted by the time they go to bed.

How the town of Ranomafana has come to link the lives of illiterate forest farmers in the small villages of southeastern Madagascar to the cities of Antananarivo, USAID's Washington, D.C., and the World Bank's Geneva, is a story of an ever-changing past. And it is to that past we now turn, as we consider how it was that the forests of Madagascar came to be home to the people of the forest, and how their forest home has come to be considered a rich possession of the globe.

In the following two chapters, I present an historical analysis of land tenure and social changes in Madagascar to bring into question how ideas of "tradition" and "custom" as something fixed in time and definitive of indigenous peoples, were applied to the Malagasy. An historical portrait of a nation and region is also useful because it shows ways in which contemporary social policies are perceived by many indigenous people as ongoing strategies to seize land and wealth, control the lives and bodies of the poor, and impose unfamiliar values and practices on local cultures and societies.

Chapter 4

No Other Place on Earth: The Historical Context of Environmental Change in Madagascar

I once described Madagascar as looking like a badly presented omelette, lying in the Indian Ocean off Africa's eastern flank, from which it was wrenched millions of years ago. Like all the best omelettes, well or badly presented, it is stuffed with goodies. The fourth largest island in the world, ninety per cent of its flora and fauna is found nowhere else. Africa is home to one species of pot-bellied baobab tree, Madagascar boasts seven. Madagascar is home to two-thirds of all the world's chameleons, from ones the size of a matchstick to ones almost as long as your arm. And so it goes on, until you become bewildered by the rich biological bounty of the island. It is a treasure trove and, if the mysterious forests are left intact and explored carefully, new and astonishing species are still to be found. Inhabited by wonderful, friendly people, it is a beautiful country, stretching its languid thousand-mile length in blue waters teeming with fish and multicoloured coral reefs. Its forests encompass everything from thick tropical to montane, to dry deciduous forest, to spiny forest as prickly as a hedgehog, and to pygmy forests only six inches high. It has lemurs as big as a four-year-old child and others that are small enough to fit into a coffee cup. It has woodlice the size of golf balls and moths the size of Regency fans. When you go on an expedition such as ours, it behooves you to keep your objectives sternly in mind, lest you be distracted and led astray by the fascinations that envelop you (Durrell 1992:5).

As this colorful—and blandly typical—introductory paragraph to a popular travel book suggests, the island of Madagascar is known more for its biodiversity of flora and fauna than for its nearly fifteen million men, women, and children who live and work amidst this biodiversity. But despite its abundance of natural resources, attracting hoards of experts, consultants, tourists, and photographers, Madagascar remains one of the poorest countries in the world, with a per capita income of approximately $235 in 1995, having fallen forty percent since the mid-seventies (World Bank 1996). The World Bank (1996:5) estimates that 74 percent of the population lives below the poverty line, and among these poor, 92 percent live in rural areas. UNICEF (1992) indicates that Madagascar is among the fifteen poorest nations in the world, with the people who live in the southeastern rainforest region where this study takes place, having the lowest average rural income in the country.

Contact with international markets has characterized Madagascar since its founding by humans. The island was first settled by both Indonesian and East African seafarers probably around 600AD (Verin 1986). Its strategic location in the Indian Ocean attracted the attention of Portuguese, Arab, Asian, British, and French traders. Throughout its history of human habitation and economic development, it has been characterized by international trade and agricultural production. While its geographic beauty has always been among the virtues noted by foreign explorers, traders, and missionaries, in the last decade the island's geography and natural resources have gained such international stature that the environment is regarded as a "global" resource meriting management by the world's major economic powers. In order to understand these contemporary issues regarding the "ancestral" lands of the forest, and ultimately, how illness is treated, it is important to understand how people came to live in the forest in the first place and how the surrounding land became cast as ancestral.

The Rise of a Pre-Colonial Autocracy

Madagascar's biological isolation has never been matched with a comparable social isolation. Indeed, its strategic position in the Indian Ocean made it a popular post for international trade not only in spices dating from the sixteenth century, but also in guns, ammunition and slaves, which were commodities traded with Europeans and mainland Africans from the eighteenth to the nineteenth centuries. The European expansion of economic trade in the Indian Ocean, dominated by a thriving slave trade between the Mascarene Islands and Madagascar, resulted in social and political changes in the rural interior as people were displaced, local economies unbalanced, and people impoverished (Larson 2000). While the effects of this trade were uneven throughout the island, the economic benefits reaching the interior contributed to the rise of a pre-colonial autocracy which shaped concepts of ethnic identity, radically altered gender relations, led to illness, malnutrition and death among large sectors of the population, and brought with it migration, industrialization and changes in agricultural production that drastically and unevenly changed the island's ecology (Larson 1992; 2000). These social forces were intensified with the imposition of colonial policies and have been replicated in many ways by recent conservation and development initiatives.

The rise of the pre-colonial Merina autocracy dates to the late-eighteenth century when the ruler of a petty kingdom, Andrianampoinimerina, seized control of the central highlands. While Andrianampoinimerina is popularly revered throughout highland Madagascar as a benevolent and sagacious ruler who centralized power during the period of anarchy associated with the international slave trade, the history of his reign presents a very different portrait. He gained power by bribing his enemies' supporters, accusing wealthy landowners of sorcery and subsequently appropriating their property, and threatening those who did not support him with slavery, imprisonment, or death (Lord 1900). Slaves were essential to his power base because they were not only economically valuable, they were also necessary to construct the kingdom and develop a domestic infrastructure (Larson 1992).

Andrianampoinimerina amassed slaves by waging attacks against villages weakened by smallpox, establishing a penal code in which transgressors were sold into slavery, and instituting taxes enabling him to seize not just the property of debtors, but the debtors themselves.[1] By exporting slaves, he was able to gain sophisticated weaponry from the British and French, which facilitated the expansion of his kingdom and helped him to establish an army (staffed through the forced military service of young men) (Bloch 1986; Larson 2000). Despite the effectiveness of these policies in bringing him to power, he was never able to rule more than one-third of the island, as the majority of the population forcefully resisted the policies and ideology he enforced (Covell 1987; Larson 1992). The resistance to the autocratic rule of the highland monarchy persists to this day and underlies much of the resistance to contemporary social policies (Allen 1995), although this resistance cannot be understood in simple ethnic terms. As Covell (1987:13) explains:

> The distinction between Merina and *côtier* [coastal people] (many of whom do not live anywhere near a coast) is the result of the existence and politics of the Merina empire, the dif-

---

1. While taxation and forced labor had been employed before Andrianampoinimerina, he escalated their practice to an unparalleled extreme (Bloch 1986:14).

ferential distribution of education that dates from imperial times, and the policies of the colonial regime and its successor government who tried to mobilize support by portraying themselves as defenders against 'Merina domination'. The conflict cannot be reduced either to ethnic or class competition, but has elements of both.

Nonetheless, the reorganization of the land and people under Andrianampoinimerina and his successors, and which was closely tied to constructions of ethnic identity, has had lasting repercussions throughout the island, and has come to be internalized in multiple ways for all of Madagascar's peoples.

Land Reorganization

The Merina kingdom emerged in association with the international trade in humans and was made possible by warfare, taxation and a penal code (Bloch 1986; Larson 2000). Warfare, directed to the forested areas of the east, increased the territory under control of Andrianampoinimerina, while taxation enlarged the royal coffers. Both had devastating effects on economies and social organizations throughout the island as people were pushed onto more marginal farming areas, women's agricultural and work responsibilities increased with the loss of men to slavery and military service, and the majority of people were dispossessed of their land (Larson 2000). But it was the establishment of a penal code directed at land reorganization, and especially crucial to the expansion of the kingdom, that most decisively altered the Malagasy social system, as well as agricultural practices (Berthier 1930; Thébault 1951).

According to Linton (1933), in his study of the southeastern Tanala social structure prior to the rise of the Merina autocracy, individual ownership of land had been unnecessary.[2] Individual ownership, to the extent land could be so conceived, was vested in the village. While there were defined boundaries, these boundaries were usually natural ones, such as rivers

---

2. Whereas Linton was specifically referring to the period prior to colonization, a review of the land tenure laws as outlined by Berthier (1930), Compte (1963), and Thébault (1951) suggests that the pattern of communal land holdings to which Linton refers had transformed during the early reigns of Andrianampoinimerina and Radama I (ca 1796-1828). It is likely, however, that the Tanala retained many of their customary practices pertaining to land tenure throughout the Merina reign (indeed, as will be discussed subsequently, resistance to land appropriation continues among the Tanala to this day).

or mountain ranges. Transgressing these boundaries by pasturing cattle or cutting *tavy* [swidden rice cultivation] could lead to war. Fallow land and virgin jungle, Linton maintained, were regarded as common property. Villagers were permitted to set traps and beehives, use timber, and gather forest products on such land. As such, it is plausible that the communal land tenure system had served to limit forest exploitation, while maintaining land rights.

Selling land outside the lineage was sanctioned only when a member of a lineage had been enslaved and money was needed for ransom. Even in this case, Linton pointed out, sale was usually regarded only as a pledge for a loan.[3] The cultural restrictions governing use of the communal land thus served to preserve biological resources, rather than enable their exploitation.

By the turn of the eighteenth century, Andrianampoinimerina's rule changed many of these practices. He began by declaring himself the proprietor of the earth (a concept later reaffirmed by all of his pre-colonial successors), in which the land was his alone (Berthier 1930).[4] Having achieved the subjugation of most of the highlands, he rewarded those who had supported him with gifts of land and administrative positions, and he used land reorganization to extend his domain. Each of his subjects, Thébault (1951:210) reported, was given an area to maintain (but not own[5]), in exchange for cattle and money. Next, he divided the land into six states, or "tribes," over which he reigned.

Each "tribe" thus created, was proprietor of the soil which was consequently assigned to it, and these lands took the generic name of *tanim-pirenara*. The *tanim-pirenara* were shared among the diverse *fokonolona* [a line of descent arising from the same ancestor, whose tomb constitutes the symbolic property around with the group is united[6]]. To demarcate property limits and avoid future disputes, a border of stones (*orimbao*)

---

3. Of course, Linton's (1933) description of land tenure was limited to the Tanala Menabe (a sub-group of the Tanala), so it cannot necessarily be extended to the whole of Madagascar, but it does provide a certain perspective on how land had been organized in the southeast, at least in one forest region.

4. Verín (1990) reported that Andrianampoinimerina was not the first king to declare the earth his own, but he was certainly the most successful (pre-colonial) ruler in the effort.

5. Ownership was acquired in other ways, as detailed subsequently.

6. What remains uncertain is when the *fokonolona* first appeared. Beaujard (1983) indicates that the *fokonolona* originated in the eastern Tanala regions in the seventeenth century, whereas Larson (1992) argues that it was the Merina king Andrianampoinimerina, who first instituted the *fokonolona* in order to diminish the power of the ruling *mpanjaka* in favor of a local control that was less threatening to Merina expansion.

was solemnly put into place around each *tanim-pirenara*. This done, within each "tribe" the *fokonolona* was provided with a portion of the land, which was shared among the families of the tribe (Thébault 1951:210). A family did not necessarily have a life-interest in the land; the *fokonolona* remained the acting proprietor and could reclaim the land at any time, while Andrianampoinimerina could reclaim the land from the *fokonolona* at any time.

To facilitate his economic goals, the new king declared that the rice fields would be shared by the various *fokonolona*, by dividing them into what were called *hetra* (Thébault 1951). The *hetra* was the collective property of the tribe or the *fokonolona*, who were responsible for collecting individual taxes on each lot (indeed, the word *hetra* has come to mean taxes in the contemporary Malagasy language). While an individual did not retain legal possession of the *hetra* rice fields, he could transfer the rights to this land to his children through succession, inheritance, or purchase. If a member of a *fokonolona* did not have a *hetra*, the *hetra* could be reclaimed and given to them. If someone died intestate, or left the tribe, the *hetra* could be reclaimed and redistributed among the tribe. Property other than rice fields was also divided similarly, and land for building houses or growing other crops was divided into *zara-tany* (literally, a division of land).

There were four ways to acquire *hetra*. Thébault (1951) indicated that the modes of acquisition and transmission of the newly created private property, included *tany vidina* (land acquired by purchase), *tanin-drazana* (patrimonial land which was transmitted by succession or inheritance), *fehivava* (land given in payment of a debt), and *lolombintany* (land granted by a royal [Andriana] chief or sovereign, for services rendered). This last form of land transfer became a common form of payment to soldiers whose service attracted the attention of the king, or to other loyal supporters of his new society. Such *lolombintany* lands, in which title was complete and without restrictions, were not subject to the *fokonolona* management, or to taxes. Moreover, the *lolombintany* was the only class of land which constituted legal possession (Thébault 1951). All other land holdings remained limited to rights to use.

Berthier (1930) suggested that these *lolombintany* lands constituted the first form of private property. The emergence of private property was not, however, a well-defined turn of events. Rather, it was a process which began before Andrianampoinimerina's reign, and outside the highlands. Certainly, the seizure of land by sixteenth and seventeenth century rulers (such as that practiced by the Antemoro and the Sakalava who forced their subjects to labor the land as serfs) constituted a form of privatizing the commons for their own benefit. Also, the exchange of land for slave ransom suggested that lineages were involuntarily relinquishing their land to others.

Dubois (1938) had further pointed out that the very annexing of land and requiring people to remain stationary were, in effect, a privatization of land that had formerly been communal. The *lolombintany*, however, did establish a definitive title to land that contributed to the growing class formation, in which certain groups were privileged over others in their access to land and resources, a process discussed in Chapter Five.

Industrialization and Environmental Change

To enforce tax collection and ensure the rapid appropriation of labor, the king prohibited geographical mobility, requiring everyone to live among what he popularized as "ancestral lands," (discussed in the following chapter) and he regulated the sale of *hetra* so that they could not pass outside the "ancestral group" or to those people now regarded as slaves (Campbell 1985; Compte 1963; Larson 1992). Although most people resisted permanent occupation of lands, and migratory lifestyles associated with shifting cultivation continued to be covertly practiced throughout the island, for those who did willingly or unwillingly settle in stationary villages, their acquiescence to state policy contributed to agricultural decline. By forcing permanent land occupation, the fallow period necessary to restore soil nutrients was shortened, and the damaging effects of shifting cultivation intensified.

By fixing people in permanent settlements, however, the Merina state was faced with the problem of ensuring that those who lived amongst the island's resources could not claim control over them. To limit local control over resources, it was necessary for the state to assert proprietorship. This was done through *terres lavavolo*. Land which was not allocated as *hetra*, or otherwise transferred as outlined above, was classified as *terres lavavolo*, or vacant land (Berthier 1930). The *lavavolo* lands, which included the forests, swamps, rivers, lakes, grasslands, and any other unoccupied land, belonged to the king. Even the earth underneath occupied land was declared property of the king—thus Andrianampoinimerina bestowed upon himself mining rights. Because cultivation of land could imply occupation, Andrianampoinimerina banned the planting of trees on hillside land in order to assure that wealthy individuals did not accumulate land by developing it (Larson 1992). In so doing, indigenous methods of forest renewal were curtailed.

While Berthier (1930) maintained that the *fokonolona* continued to enjoy the privilege of using the forests and pastures, Tacchi (1892) indicated that one of the first things Andrianampoinimerina did upon his rise to power was to promulgate strict laws concerning the forest. These laws prohibited anyone from taking any firewood, upon the penalty of one dollar and one bullock.[6] The discrepancy between Berthier's argument that communal use of the forests was permitted, and Tacchi's assertion that it was strictly forbidden, is probably explained by regional and temporal differences, in which certain customary practices continued without sanction in some regions or during some periods, but new decrees were more strictly enforced in others, particularly if the forest area was of value to the monarchy.

The value of the forests to the monarchy was considerable. Although Andrianampoinimerina's reign never extended to the southeastern forests that comprise the Ranomafana region, his land policies did have significant impact on the forested terrain of the highlands, and his social policies fostered considerable migration into the southeastern forests. Several authors have pointed to the magnitude of forest destruction during the development of the Merina empire (e.g., Boiteau 1982; Verín 1990; Tacchi 1892). In order to build up the empire and promote international trade, a massive industrialization crusade using forced labor was initiated under Andrianampoinimerina; it included construction of a massive hydraulics system, as well as roads and railways from Antananarivo to the eastern coast. These projects, which continued during the reign of Andrianampoinimerina's successors Radama I and Ranavalona I, destroyed enormous expanses of forests, particularly from the capitol city of Antananarivo in the central highlands, to the eastern port of Tamatave on the coast. Indeed, Bloch (1989), Hardenbergh (1992), and Verín (1986), have suggested that the Merina expansion and development of waterworks caused total deforestation throughout much of the eastern forests in this region.[7]

The mechanisms employed by Malagasy rulers to advance the social transformation they envisioned included labor appropriation, land reorganization, economic restructuring, taxation, and social reorganization; moreover, the European demand for slaves in the Mascarene Islands led to an increase in warfare (aimed at taking captives who could be commodified (Bloch 1986; Campbell 1985; Larson 1992; 2000). Profits from these slave raids were then used to facilitate political ambitions rather than economic development. A wealthy elite thus emerged, along with an impoverished majority. These mechanisms of economic and political re-

---

6. The only exception to this rule, Tacchi wrote, was when a woman gave birth to a child, because it was the custom to place the mother and child beside a very large fire.

7. To this day, the long-term effects of this destruction are readily apparent from the eroded hillsides which flank the roads from the capitol to the eastern coasts. The dry and fissured earth is commonly photographed to show the effects of deforestation from *tavy*, with no reference ever made to the role the roadways (now paved highways) played in creating this damaged landscape.

structuring by the Malagasy Merina were echoed by foreign powers in the nineteenth century, as they united with the highland elite in an effort to lay the foundation for colonial rule,[8] and subsequently by the Social Democratic Party (PSD) of Philip Tsiranana immediately following independence (Allen 1995).[9]

While there was considerable resistance to Merina rule, open resistance led to public persecution, incarceration or death. Thus, covert resistance became commonplace. The primary form of covert resistance was to relocate to deeply forested lands, particularly the southeastern forests, where the new laws of the Merina kingdom were unenforceable. Such relocation, however, had serious costs. Malaria was far more prevalent, and the lands were less fertile. But even the minimal existence afforded by living in these steep and densely forested terrains provided many with a greater chance at survival than they would have under servitude to the Merina kingdom.

One reason resistance to Merina rule was so great was that it included forced labor and military conscription. Soldiers and civilians could be called to duty on a moment's notice, regardless of their agricultural obligations. In a letter to his wife, the Rev. Griffiths wrote:

> All the people of the inland provinces, and on the eastern coast from Vohimarina to Fort Dauphin, have not a week that they can call their own to cultivate their ground or provide for their families, but are required to engage in some government service or other, as tilling the ground, felling timber, making and carrying charcoal, collecting wax and gum copal, etc. and carrying hides from the interior to Tamatave. All the tailors have their service exacted in the same manner by the Government without any remuneration. The people often remark, with feelings of stoical indifference, "We shall not teach our children *anything*, for the more they know, the harder will be their service" (Griffiths 1840 in Cousins 1895:344, emphasis in original).

---

8. Although the French appealed to anti-Merina sentiments in an effort to disempower the Merina and gain support throughout the island, they found themselves aligning with the educated elite of the country who were better able to provide administrative support to the government. Nonetheless, the Merina were in the forefront of the resistance movement against the French as they found their own power diminishing (Allen 1995; Covell 1987).

9. The PSD party continued to promote highlander/coastal or Merina/non-Merina divisions as central to its nationalist policies, while at the same time it exacerbated class divisions between the urban elites and the rural peasantry as it prospered under the Merina elite (Bloch 1986:33).

Following Andrianampoinimerina's death in 1810, a succession of his descendants and their spouses ruled the island, none more oppressive than Queen Ranavalona, whose open hostility to Europeans was matched only by her cruelty to her own subjects, a cruelty so great and unforgiving that it has been celebrated in fiction through the historical adventures of "Flashman," in which author George MacDonald Fraser (1988:246) describes her in the following imaginary detail:

> I've seen her, leaning on that verandah, with her creatures about her, gazing down on the scene below; the ring of Hova guardsmen, the circle of torches flaming over the archways, the huddled groups of unfortunates, male and female, from mere striplings to old decrepit folk, cowering and waiting. They might be recaptured slaves, or fugitives hunted out of the forests and mountains, or criminals, or non-Hova tribesmen, or suspected Christians, or anyone who, under her tyranny, had merited punishment. She would look down for a long time, and then nod at one group and grunt: "Burning," and then at another "Crucifixion," and at a third, "Boiling." And so on, through the ghastly list—starvation, or flaying alive, or dismembering, or whatever horror occurred to her monstrous taste. Then she would go inside—and next day the sentences would be carried out at Ambohipotsy in front of a cheering mob. Sometimes she attended herself, watching unmoved, and then going home to the palace to spend hours praying to her personal idols under the paintings in her reception room.

Although MacDonald's account is a fabricated one, it nonetheless draws on both myth and history to illustrate the ways in which the Queen's sadistic rule led to the popular acceptance of foreign domination as an alternative to her tyranny. And while accounts of her reign are peppered with images of her tossing Christians over cliffs in an effort to cleanse the island of foreign influence, Queen Ranavalona was ultimately responsible for formalizing relations between the Malagasy state and European powers, as the British and French competed for control of the island during the early nineteenth century (a competition that endured throughout the century) (Bloch 1986). Fearing an alliance between the British and French, whose combined power could easily crush her government, along with a growing dependence on the military, industrial and administrative resources of the Europeans, Queen Ranavalona established formal ties with the European government. This move, which was supported by the majority of the populace, who viewed European authority as preferable to the cruelty of the queen's command (Bloch 1986).

The French government seized upon the instability and social inequalities associated with the Merina monarchy by appealing to the population and alleging that they would represent the interests of rural and coastal Malagasy whose non-Merina identity rendered them, the majority, socially marginal.[10] At the same time, the newly-formed highland elite, who had been rewarded with European educations for their support of the monarchy, were advantageously positioned for key administrative positions in the new colonial state.

By the second half of the nineteenth century, the Europeans were to position themselves in the Merina kingdom and Malagasy society so firmly that their colonial designs were effortlessly installed. Their policies of land and labor appropriation differed very little from that of the Merina, but through their military and economic strength, and assisted by the infrastructure that the Merina monarchs had begun to set into place, they were able to seize the land and its resources on an even larger scale.

Colonial Land and Labor Policies

The colonial era, from 1895 to 1960, was marked by forced labor, land appropriation, taxation, the introduction of cash crops, forest conservation, and the development of a medical infrastructure.

Labor was controlled through laws (passed in 1897, 1902, and 1907) requiring all adult men, ages 16 to 60, to work 50 days a year for the colonial government, without pay, and to pay a head tax of 2.50 FF (Hanson 1997).

> In general, throughout the first three decades of the 20th century, the French colonial administration ransacked the eastern forests for cash and labor. These revenues, rather than being returned to the region via meaningful development projects, were employed either to pay off the rather large debt and fines the pre-colonial state had incurred to France (Rabearimanana 1985:317), or invested in the *colons* (Fremigacci 1986:327). Taxes on the common people proved inordinately high. For example, taken together, the various forms of taxes owed to the administration by the average household in 1918 reached 26.60FF (ibid: 303). Simply unable to pay this amount, individuals were forced to take out loans and/or labor for the administration (Hanson 1997:67,68).

Taxation, however, required a stationary population. Jarosz (1993:373) indicates that *tavy* was incompatible with colonial objectives because swid-

---

10. French rule was further assured, as European powers negotiated among themselves for control over African lands, with Great Britain ceding an interest in Madagascar in favor of control over the island of Zanzibar.

den rice farmers tended to live in scattered, extended family groups which moved frequently. Tax collection and labor appropriation (for forced labor parties) were difficult to carry out in communities practicing *tavy*, because those who practiced it moved frequently. Consequently, laws prohibiting the burning of forest cover and regenerating growth were enacted in 1881 (by the Merina autocracy, toward the same ends), and in 1900 and 1902 by the French colonial state. In 1900, the *Service Forestier* was established, with authority to grant forest concessions and enforce rules regulating use of forest resources. In 1913, the Governor General of the colonial state assumed authority over all forest concessions of 100 hectares or more, and in that same year, *tavy* was prohibited throughout the island and linked to the prohibition was the promotion of irrigated rice agriculture, which was considered more sustainable and intensive. By prohibiting *tavy*, the state not only sought to facilitate tax collection as people were fixed into stationary settlements, but they also wanted to protect forest resources for commodification by the state and European mining and timber concessions. The practice continued, however, particularly in the southeastern forests where swidden agriculture was the most efficient and productive way to farm such steep terrain. As such, in 1930 the Governor General was granted authority over all permits to use forest resources, and punishments, including fines and imprisonment, were established for transgressors. Hanson (1997:78) points out that these decrees were largely aimed at French concessionaires who exploited the "principle forest products" of ebony, wood for industrial use, charcoal, and bark for textiles and fibers. While the ban on *tavy* was directed toward the rural Malagasy farmer, the regulations regarding forest exploitation were intended to facilitate and regulate exploitation of the forest for European industrialists.

Another major feature of colonial forest policies came in 1928, when one million hectares of forests were divided into nine separate reserves and redefined as "protected" areas (Hanson 1997). In so doing, the prohibition of *tavy* was linked to the enclosure of forests for conservation purposes at the same time that exploitation of these same forests was facilitated by laws regulating and sanctioning the use of the forest for industrial development. The southeastern forests were especially productive for European industrialists as timber operations and coffee plantations were launched concurrently with the prohibition on *tavy*. It is no surprise, then, that *tavy* became, once again, a covert act: as during the reign of Andrianampoinimerina, *tavy* became a practice embedded not just in the symbolic realm of the ancestors, it came to represent resistance for those people whose economic livelihoods had been dependent upon shifting cultivation (see Hanson 1997 on *tavy* as a form of resistance).

Jarosz (1993) indicates that the colonial policy promoting irrigated agriculture in place of *tavy* failed because the regional variations of the island were not uniformly conducive to wet-rice irrigation. In those highland areas where suitable flat-lands made irrigated rice production feasible, the ban was effective, but in mountainous areas, such as the eastern coastal forests, enforcing the ban was impossible as farmers continued to practice *tavy*—the only possible way to grow rice in those regions.

Jarosz (1993:374) further suggests that the failure of the ban on *tavy* was in part due to the resistance of farmers who interpreted the colonial policy in differing ways:

> Peasants interpreted the ban as a form of labor control compelling them to work for wages and buy rice, thus losing their independence. Moreover, the ban meant that the sacred space where the living engaged in dialogue with the ancestors was annihilated by colonial decree. Mass revolts and resistance, as well as scattered, individual acts of noncompliance, spoke directly to this annihilation and the divergent meanings of *tavy* to the Malagasy peasants and the state.

One additional reason the prohibition on *tavy* failed could be attributed to the hypocrisy many Malagasy felt was reflected in the policy. Jarosz (1993) points out that *tavy* was portrayed as environmentally destructive, while at the same time forest resources were viewed as resources of value to outsiders, a discourse she indicates resembles academic discourse on the subject:

> Early academic accounts of shifting cultivation characterize it as unplanned, aimless, nomadic, unproductive, and uneconomical in the utilization of land and labor and destructive of the environment (Whittlesey 1937). The discourse of colonial conservation parallels the academic view. Writing about the forests of Madagascar in 1890, one observer on a missionary tour expressed "a hope that the present wholesale destruction of the forest by the natives may be soon effectually stopped by the Government, and that its valuable resources may be speedily utilized" (Baron 1890, 211 in Jarosz 1993:372).

Another major agricultural innovation coincided with the promotion of irrigated rice production and the prohibition against *tavy*, and that was the introduction of cash crops. In the southeastern forests, this production was primarily in coffee, but banana trees were also planted for export. Jarosz (1993:370,371) indicates that export production varied regionally, but that the introduction of coffee crops in the southeastern forests was especially destructive of the forest ecology:

> According to Temple (1972), the soil erosion rates on coffee plots are nearly double those of subsistence plots, because broad

expanses of bare soil under the coffee bushes are particularly vul-
nerable to violent storms during the rainy season. The state's
emphasis on export production led to a pattern of uneven economic development and regional fragmentation (Isnard 1971;
Hugon 1987) which created increasing production pressures
and demands upon environmental resources.

The introduction of coffee cultivation also led to shortfalls in
rice production. Razoharinoro-Randriamboavonjy (1971), Al-
thabe (1982), and Rakotoarisoa and Richard (1987) have noted
the tension between cash cropping and rainfed rice regimes in
terms of claims on land and labor time. Due to its labor demands and attractive producer prices, coffee cultivation increased in popularity among European settlers and Malagasy
farmers. As rainfed fields were abandoned—the causalities of
labor shortfalls, low producer prices, cyclones, and drought—
food security in the eastern region was eroded.

In the 1930s and 1940s, coffee plantations, having been introduced in
Madagascar in the 1920s, were expanded in the southeastern forests, and
area *colons* [colonial officers] were granted free access to appropriate lands
for such production (Hanson 1997). Hanson (1997:70,71) discusses how
the introduction of cash-crop production, in association with the shift to
irrigated rice production, affected the farmers of the southeastern Ranomafana region:

> ...beginning in the early 1900's, French authorities forced the
> Tanala to abandon their mountaintop homes and settle the val-
> ley spaces along the major roadways. The motivations behind
> these dislocations were diverse. However, in the Ranomafana
> region, the goal of the colonial administration was particularly
> clear. During the first decades of the twentieth century, then
> Governor General Marcel Olivier laid the fiscal basis for the
> development of coffee plantations in the region. Olivier un-
> derstood that to secure the labor force needed for these plan-
> tations, he would first have to force the Tanala to settle the val-
> ley floors, and second, introduce irrigated rice culture to keep
> the population fed.

As the coffee trees matured, however, they became less productive. This
decline in cash-crop production, accompanied by less investment in subsistence agriculture, contributed to rice-shortages and economic decline
in the mid-1940s. The people living in the southeastern forests, having already had a history of resistance to Merina rule, were among those most
affected by the colonial policies of forced labor and land appropriation

(Covell 1987); consequently, they came to be in the forefront of resistance to colonial rule (Covell 1987). Thus, it is not surprising that in 1947, an indigenous resistance movement emerged from the eastern forested regions near Ifanadiana, a movement that was to become one of the most devastating of colonial rebellions. More than 100,000 Malagasy died in their ineffective efforts to gain independence from colonial rule, when Senegalese men were brought to Madagascar to serve the French army and kill their African counterparts (Allen 1995; Mannoni 1990). Allen (1995:47) describes the colonial repression which followed as "one of the most bloody acts of repression in colonial history," and included execution, torture, starvation, and banishment into the desert, as among the tactics the colonial administration employed to suppress the insurrection. The post-rebellion period, lasting until 1956, included a complex propaganda campaign in which French sympathizers were repatriated, convicted conspirators were executed, and all news reporting the events was censured. The result of these responses was that the rebellion of 1947 was rapidly mythologized by both the colonial state and by the diverse Malagasy themselves.

In the southeastern forests of Madagascar, where the rebellion was the most violent and the suppression the most severe (Covell 1987), the rebellion symbolizes the unity of the "people of the forest" in their defiance of foreign control over their land and livelihoods, and their victimization by these same policies and the oppression which ensued. At the same time, memories of the period conflict, revealing that social differences do indeed contribute to differing memories. For example, while discussing the experience of the rebellion with residents of Ranotsara, two village elders provide telling accounts of how men and women were differently affected. Masobe, originally from an eastern coastal village, and his wife Tody, lived in Ranomafana from the late 1940s until the 1960s, where Masobe worked as a cook in the local hotel, and Tody, close to her home village of Ranotsara, farmed the *tavy* fields she had inherited from her family. He describes the infamous year of 1947, when all of the eastern forests were colonial battlegrounds. "The men went to the deepest parts of the forest to watch the villages from a distance, to see if the soldiers had arrived. The *vazaha* [colonial administration] had brought Senegalese soldiers to the area to chase us into Ranomafana, where we could be guarded. Men were forced to work for the *vazaha*. Women were not always strong enough to go with us into the forest, and so they stayed in the village"

Nirina is in her late seventies or eighties; her grandfather was one of the founders of the village of Ranotsara, and her husband of fifty years, Faly, was a local *mpanjaka* [indigenous leader]. She remembers this period well. "Masobe said women were not strong enough to go to the forest? What does he know! It was hardest on women because we had to do our own work *and* the men's work. We had to grow rice, and take it to the men. We also had to teach girls and boys work they did not do before." For example, she indicated that boys had to learn to cook, and girls had to learn to chop wood. "What can Masobe know of women's work!?" Nirina asked rhetorically.

Masobe, however, argued that men would come down at night to tend the crops, or they began cultivating in the forest. Both agreed that these years were hard on everybody, and the violence they witnessed left deep impressions on their hearts that outsiders often fail to recognize when telling the farmers what, and how, and where, to grow their crops.

Population Migration and Land Reorganization in the Ranomafana/Ifanadiana Region

As this chapter has shown, the southeastern forests of Madagascar have provided a refuge from control and domination for the last two hundred years. Originally founded between the twelfth and fourteenth centuries by entrepreneurs seeking to capitalize on international trade on the eastern coast, the area that is now known as the Ranomafana/Ifanadiana region was a safe haven for cattle thieves and slave traders, who obtained much of their stock from the western regions south of the expanding Merina kingdom, a region which later became the administrative division of the Betsileo. Kottak (1971a:14) notes that slaves were exchanged for firearms, and that this exchange contributed to the concept of a Tanala ethnicity (discussed in more detail in the following chapter), as military coordinators and those who headed raiding parties gathered on fortified hills and used their firearms to gain power.

By the eighteenth century another wave of immigrants came to the region. Hanson discusses these waves of immigration in the Ranomafana region:

> It is important to distinguish the waves of refugees to the Ranomafana forests...from a set of more organized and larger-scale immigrations from the north which occurred between the 18th and 19th centuries. Most of these latter newcomers were of Betsileo origin, escaping their highland homes in fear of forced labor and taxes, and seeking the more fertile soils of the Ranomafana forests. Solondraibe (1986:152) speaks of two mass Betsileo immigrations. The first resulted from the arduous demands issuing from the Betsileo kingdoms of Lalangina and Isandra; the second, from similar demands of the Merina kings

Andrianampoinimerina and Radama I. It is, for the most part, these latter two groups of immigrants who founded the villages now surrounding the RNP [Ranomafana National Park] and whose descendants participate in the RNPP [Ranomafana National Park Project]. A final group to arrive near the Ranomafana region during the pre-colonial period was part of what Campbell (1988) calls the "Merina colonies". These "colonies" were settlements of civilians and military officers sent from the high plateau to found agricultural communities. These "communities," however, also became collection points for the slave trade. The effects of these garrisons on the eastern forest cover is significant (Hanson 1997:58,59).

Thus establishing themselves amongst the slave traders and cattle thieves, the new settlers themselves became "people of the forest," or "Tanala."

Another wave of immigrants, coming from highland urban areas, settled during the 1920s and 1930s, when coffee and timber concessions were introduced. This group of people came to benefit from economic opportunities associated with the expanding market economy and settled along major transportation routes of Ranomafana-Ifanadiana-Mananjary trail or the newly-constructed National Route 25. Merchants followed, "seeking to develop businesses along the roadways. These peoples were of Malagasy, French, Chinese and Indo-Pakistani origins. They established coffee plantations, set-up small shops featuring local forest products, and operated lumber concessions" (Hanson 1997:60). At the same time as these outside entrepreneurial groups were settling, colonial officials encouraged the already settled highland farmers to labor for hire on wet rice fields in the valleys.

Coinciding with the establishment of the colonial state in Madagascar, and the penetration of its agricultural and forestry policies into the southeastern regions, another change was underway. According to local legend, at the end of the nineteenth century a thermal hot springs had been discovered in the southeastern forest region of Madagascar. By the 1940s, this discovery led to the transformation of the village that was then termed Vatomainty ["black stone"] into a celebrated resort for medical treatment and cure. A multitude of healers and chronically ill people migrated to the area throughout the first part of the twentieth century, and by mid-century, Vatomainty was renamed Ranomafana ("hot water"). Throughout the period of colonial occupation, Ranomafana was popular as a resort town, renown for the healing properties of its waters, and frequented by European and elite Malagasy from urban areas, while the surrounding rural communities remained dependent on subsistence farming.

Thus, the forests of southeastern Madagascar, presently characterized by conservation and development discourse as representing an intact ecosystem threatened by the spread of *tavy* fires, whose only social context is regarded as, at best, rooted in poverty, poor technology, and high birth rates (e.g. Harrison 1992; Jolly 1987; Keck, Sharma and Feder 1994; Pryor 1990; World Bank 1994) or attributed to ethnic tradition, at worst (RNPP 1994) have, in fact, been farmed and protected by forest residents both acquiescing to, and resisting, state and international economic policies for the last two hundred years. That the forests have survived at all, is not due to the natural processes of a virgin ecosystem naturally and harmoniously flourishing beyond the reach of humans. The forests have, in fact, been home to humans who have variously preserved the forest cover for protection and concealment (Hanson 1997; Kottak 1971); and been forced to burn it for production of cash crops (Jarosz 1993). Moreover, the economic pressures brought on by the pre-colonial and colonial states likely had repercussions for the forest cover because many subsistence farmers would have been forced to intensify production and limit fallow to pay taxes and crops to both pre-colonial and colonial authorities, and been induced to increase shifting cultivation to offset the social and economic repercussions of forced labor. Many of these same policies (such as bans on *tavy*, imposition of taxes and fines, and encouragement of cash-crop production) have been reproduced by state and international policies since colonization. Nonetheless, these historical circumstances, linked in many respects to broader global processes of economic development, are never fully implicated in the accounts policy makers put forth to explain the vast ecological degradation unfolding in Madagascar. Moreover, the role that development itself plays in the over-utilization of environmental resources is similarly omitted from most international conservation discourse. Instead, development has been presented as the salvation of the forests.

Conservation and Development: Post-Colonial Land and Economic Reforms

In 1960 Madagascar gained sovereignty, but remained dependent upon France through French control of private enterprise and the post-colonial government (with many French colonial administrators and advisors remaining in government posts). This period marked the First Republic of President Philibert Tsiranana, or the period of the Malagasy Republic (République Malgache). By 1972, Tsiranana's power declined, with a peasant rebellion and military coup culminating in the collapse of the First Republic, to be replaced by the Democratic Republic of Madagascar.

The Second Republic of Madagascar was a Soviet-styled Socialist Democracy, led by Didier Ratsiraka, from 1975 to 1991. Ratsiraka advocated an isolationist stance, rejecting all foreign-owned industries or land holdings, while maintaining political alliances with then Eastern Europe, Korea, and China. Sharp (1993:11) points out that although this period was characterized as a socialist one, "its economy may be defined more clearly as a form of state capitalism, where the ownership of all major industries and land holdings rests with the national government."

Ratsiraka's policies, however, which included several poorly designed investments in national industry, and massive investment in the urban sector with profound neglect of the rural sector, led to rising international debt. Fearing an international economic crisis should a large number of post-colonial countries default on the debts they were unable to repay, the World Bank and the International Monetary Fund (IMF) had instituted structural adjustment programs throughout the developing world. These programs were designed to facilitate debt repayment and promote the global expansion of a free market economy (Gershman and Irwin 2000). By pressuring the indebted countries to privatize the social sector (including education, social security, and health care), reducing or eliminating tariffs, government subsidies, or quotas that had limited imported goods and facilitated domestic trade, by deregulating domestic industries and services, and by devaluing local currencies, private investment in developing countries was encouraged, while investment in the social sector drastically reduced.

Faced with the heavy debts incurred in the post-colonial years, in 1980, during the Second Republic, Madagascar became the first African socialist state to agree to structural adjustment policies of the IMF. As was to become common for most post-colonial countries, the adjustments Madagascar entered into included privatization of banking and industry, and repeated devaluation of the Malagasy Franc[11] which led to 100 percent inflation.

This period, the late 1980s and early 1990s, also saw the introduction of a multitude of international conservation development projects. This is because the World Bank's agricultural reforms in Madagascar were tied to the conservation of the island's "megabiodiversity" (Allen 1995). At the same time, the United States Agency for International Development (USAID), having been empowered through the U.S. Endangered Species Act of 1976 to regulate resource use in developing countries, made Madagascar a major conservation priority. The Endangered Species Act

> ...stated that the preservation of animal and plant species through the regulation of hunting and trade, limitations on pol-

---

11. 10-15% from 1982 to 1986; 46% in 1987; and 13% in January 1991.

lution, and the protection of wildlife habitats, should be an important objective of U.S. development assistance. Protection of endangered species was also emphasized (USAID n/d:17).

USAID subsequently identified Madagascar as

one of ten "threatened hot spots": a series of tropical areas identified as being critical to the global conservation of plant and animal diversity. Because of its high levels of biodiversity and endemism, Madagascar has been termed "the single highest major conservation priority in the world" (USAID n/d:1). Madagascar is categorized as a "Group I" country, i.e., has "urgent needs for natural resource interventions" (USAID n/d:19).

Conservation was further linked to development through the United States Foreign Assistance Act (FAA), section 119, amended in 1986.

AID is required to enter into long-term arrangments in which the recipient country agrees to protect ecosystems, support research, and deny assistance for actions that significantly degrade protected areas. CDSS's [Country Development Strategy Statements] are required to include an analysis of the actions needed to conserve biological diversity. Whenever feasible, activities are to be carried out by PVO's [Private Voluntary Organizations] (USAID n/d:18).

The linking of conservation with structural adjustment reforms was institutionalized nationally through the Madagascar's 1987-88 Environmental Action Plan (EAP) (the first such environmental plan in Africa). A World Bank creation, the EAP took the position that indigenous land management practices were environmentally destructive because individuals lacked incentive to increase productivity and protect ancestral lands (Leisz, Robles and Gage 1994). This "tragedy of the commons" concept, which McCay and Acheson (1987) have shown to be fundamentally incorrect because indigenous communities may indeed have mechanisms for protecting commonly held lands, has been presumed by the World Bank to be a necessary precondition for the conservation of the island.

Inherent in the EAP is the belief that it is necessary to secure people's rights of access to their land and natural resource base in the periphery zones of Madagascar's protected areas. The 15-year, three-phase plan emphasizes that security to land is important to environmental conservation (Leisz, Robles and Gage 1994:4).

In other words, the "tragedy of the commons" presumes that communal control of land is inherently contradictory to the protection of that land, and only through private control of land will people be induced to safeguard it. Thus, World Bank programs promoting the registration of private land titles is presented as a conservation policy, rather than an economic policy.

Then in 1989 Madagascar entered into the Debt-for-Nature Swap, exchanging $2.1 million of debt for conservation projects, and another $1 million with the World Wildlife Fund. Proceeds from the trade were earmarked for national parks management, erosion control and training of park rangers (Allen 1995:177). The following year, USAID developed a program entitled SAVEM (Sustainable Approaches to Viable Environmental Management) which was "to establish sustainable human and natural ecosystems in areas of Madagascar where biodiversity was threatened" (SAVEM 1997:1).

Madagascar currently has 36 specifically defined protected areas, which include national parks, special reserves, and nature reserves, and over 260 protected areas more broadly defined to include Classified Forests and Reforestation Zones. Many of these protected areas were established during the colonial area. While Leisz, Robles and Gage (1994) suggest that during the colonial years, strict enforcement of exclusionary policies in the forests was enforced through the imposition of fines and imprisonment for anyone who transgressed the human/nature boundaries, Hanson (1997) suggests that enforcement remained uneven. Certainly during the postcolonial years prior to the EAP, strict enforcement eased up.

With the return of foreign powers safeguarding the storehouses of nature, fines and imprisonment returned as punishment to those residents who materially benefitted from the "global resources" by using them in any way. To mitigate the effects of sharply curtailing local access to the natural environment, peripheral or buffer zones were established as part of UNESCO's mid-1980's Man and Biosphere Program.

> The main objective of UNESCO's Biosphere Reserves begun in the late 1960's is to protect a core area of biodiversity and at the same time involve the surrounding human population in benefitting from the reserve through better land use practices and sustainable development activities. The reserves are designed to include different zones of human activity. At the center of the reserve is the core zone, where human activity is strictly regulated to ensure a maximum of protection to the biodiversity in the reserve. Around the core is a buffer zone where limited human activity, such as limited herding, limited agriculture, and the gathering of forest products is allowed by the forest service. Finally, around the buffer zone is the transition zone where peo-

ple live in their villages and work on their land. In the two zones where human activities are officially allowed by the state, reserve operators undertake research and extension projects which involve local inhabitants in research on better land use practices and, also, sustainable development activities (Gregg and McGean 1985; Batiss 1986) (Leisz, Robles and Gage 1994:3,4).

In order to coordinate the protected areas of Madagascar, the World Bank established the "National Association for the Management of Protected Areas" [ANGAP] in Madagascar. Funded by the World Bank and USAID, this institution serves as the Malagasy national coordinating institute of all protected areas, in conjunction with the national *Departement d'Eau et Forets* [Department of Water and Forests]. Six ANGAP protected area projects were thereby identified for SAVEM funding:

> Recognizing that these areas were being threatened, in part by deforestation and exploitation, the projects were constructed as integrated conservation and development projects (ICDP's) and based on the concept that local populations will alter their behavior (to conservation of the environment) if they see a relationship between their economic and social well being to the protected area and if they are empowered to make the right kinds of decisions....In general figures, the ICDP's received approximately eighteen and a half million dollars ($18,500,000) through SAVEM for a period of approximately 3 1/2 years (SAVEM 1997:1).

Among these Integrated Conservation and Development Projects that the United States government finances is the Ranomafana National Park Project. The Project was not, however, the first post-colonial development initiative in the region. Following independence in 1960, the next in-flux of outsiders were the Japanese, who funded the building of the JIRAMA dam on the Namorona River in Ranomafana in the early 1970s. The dam was to provide electricity to the distant city of Fianarantsoa and to a sawmill located near there, as well as to the town of Ifananadiana and the businesses and homes of newly-arrived residents of Ranomafana. Hiring local labor to provide electricity to the city of Fianarantsoa, the dam was perceived by most as a favorable project because local people were employed. When the Ranomafana National Park Project came two decades later, it was with mixed feelings. Recalling the brutality of the colonial years and the continual efforts to appropriate the forest lands of the region, outsiders were viewed as thieves. At the same time, recalling the economic opportunities of the dam, outsiders were equally perceived as cash-rich, and therefore, short-term opportunities to gain additional income were in sight for some.

As a consequence of its celebrated waters, resort ambience, and strategic location on the main highway linking the highlands to the coastal city of Mananjary, by the mid-1980s Ranomafana had become a very important market center for residents residing in the nearby forest villages, because it attracted numerous outsiders and outside money.

In the late 1980s, however, the role of Ranomafana in the lives of forest residents changed dramatically. During that time, and shortly following the drastic social and economic cut-backs associated with structural adjustment programs, a primatology research team from Duke University visited the Ranomafana region to locate and assess endangered lemur populations. Accompanied by local guides, the researchers were shown several species of lemur which live in the forests of the region. One of these, the Golden Bamboo Lemur, was unknown to Western scientists, and another, the Greater Bamboo Lemur, was believed to be extinct. Following this find by Westerners, coinciding with the 1986 U.S. Foreign Assistance Act which mandated that the United States Agency for International Development (USAID) link development aid with environmental protection, and with USAID's own declaration of Madagascar as a priority for such aid, 41,500 hectares of the local forests were declared a protected area.

And so it was that on August 14, 1990, through a grant agreement between Duke University and USAID, the Ranomafana National Park Project (RNPP) was established as the administrating agency responsible for managing social and environmental changes associated with the Ranomafana National Park, thereby becoming one of six Integrated Conservation and Development Projects (ICDP's) in Madagascar, and incorporated into USAID's Sustainable Approaches to Viable Environmental Management (SAVEM) programs.

As this chapter has shown, Malagasy forests have represented contested terrain for centuries, and traditions tied to the forest may not be so long-lived as often believed because population migrations, changing patterns of land-use, and local forms of resistance to governmental decrees have contributed to the forging of "traditions" such as *tavy*. In the following chapter, I continue this discussion of the history of Madagascar with a focus on how land and labor policies launched by Andrianampoinimerina and developed by subsequent rulers were inextricably linked to the social restructuring of the island. This social manipulation included deepening the divisions of class and caste, fundamentally altering gender relations, and creating "tribal" divisions currently conceptualized as "ethnic" ones and directly tied to concepts of race. In so doing, illness related to poverty and geographical inaccessibility became naturalized as "tropical" illness, while health care and healing became aligned with concepts of morality. By relegating the most impoverished and geographically isolated groups to an ethnic status deemed "backward," "lazy," "ignorant," and "promiscuous" (all terms I often heard used by Project management and others to describe local residents), the association between living in the forest and healing with its medicines became simplified as a "tradition" uniformly practiced by everyone so grouped.

Chapter 5

Social Status and
Access to Land

The history of land reorganization and agricultural policy in Madagascar has had profound effects on Malagasy social organization and in particular, it has been tied to changing identities. In this chapter, I focus on the history of Merina, Betsileo and Tanala ethnic identities. I then show how the Ranomafana National Park Project, in seeking to control forest resources, conflated "ethnic" identities with agricultural practices through their understandings of the concept of culture; as a result, the social relationships and historical experiences of forest farmers in southeastern Madagascar have been replaced by ethnic categories and "tradition."

The way in which ethnicity has been tied to land-use practices in Madagascar is similar to the ways in which ethnicity and land-use were represented by colonial governments in other African societies. For example, in West Africa, the persistence of ethnic stereotypes has been facilitated by local residents themselves who play on ideas of ethnicity to achieve their own political objectives.

Among the Kissidougou of Guinea, for example, Fairhead and Leach (1996) show how colonial stereotypes of ethnic differences were associated with how one interacted with the environment. People were distinguished as either "forest people" or "savanna people," ignoring the ways in which ecological knowledge and the management of local resources were shared by members of these allegedly different "ethnic" groups. Nonetheless, Fairhead and Leach (1996:118) show how the imposition of ethnicity on the Kissidougou has been reinforced by Africans themselves, as urban and rural Kissia invoke their alleged "ethnicity" in order to express solidarity as people who have a common history and "share one forest." In Fairhead's and Leach's analysis, the Kissia use concerns about the environment to raise political and cultural issues. Similar processes operate in the Ranomafana region, as I shall show, where social unity becomes expressed as a Tanala ethnicity when contrasted to outside control, yet its importance to identity and practice diminishes in the village, where lineage cleaves the community, and caste forms a nearly impenetrable boundary between economic classes.

Tribalism and Concepts
of Race in Madagascar

...one of our new friends observed that although the Malagasy do use the word "tribes" it gives *vazaha* a wrong impression. In his view this word suggests wider differences of ethnic
origin, language and custom than exist in Madagascar. He
pointed out that apart from a small Kishwahili [sic]-speaking
community of Comorians (immigrants of Afro-Shirazi stock
from the Comoro Islands), all the Malagasy speak mutually in-
telligible dialects of Malagasy and share a unique common culture. The many regional variations in custom are superficial,
based mainly on contrasting natural environments and past political divisions. They are not, he insisted, marked enough to
be properly described as *tribal* differences. I did not presume
to argue; the Malagasy are sensitive on this issue, having learned
the hard way that internal dissension invites *vazaha* intervention. They are well aware that at present both Moscow and
Washington would welcome any excuse for directly influencing political developments within Madagascar. Nevertheless,
as we traveled further and noticed the radical physical differences
between the "highland people" and the "coastal people," we decided that the use of "tribes" — however politically undesir-
able — makes ethnographic sense (Murphy 1985:107,108, emphasis in the original).

This quote, taken from a popular travel book of Madagascar, illuminates
three issues regarding the study of ethnicity in Madagascar. The first is
that Madagascar is perceived by many as divided between highland and
coastal populations and that these geographical divisions have become
cast as tribal divisions; the second is that ethnicity in Madagascar is often
conflated with race, with differences between people conceptualized less
as social differences and more as biological ones; and third, enlightenment
on the shaky ground of tribal divisions notwithstanding, old ideas die hard.
Dervla Murphy begins her narrative by disclosing that she has been told
tribalism is an historical and political construct, but concludes that because she saw *physical differences* among people, she would hold firm to
the notion that the *social grouping* of tribes make ethnographic sense.

Ethnographers and historians, however, have sought to dispel, rather
than reaffirm, the concept of natural tribal divisions (see, for example,
Bloch 1986; Kottak 1971b; Larson 1992, 2000). While Madagascar is

said to be home to eighteen different ethnic groups, historical and ethnographic analyses have shown that these ethnic groups are political and historical constructions that originated both as an expression of, and response to, the expansion of the pre-colonial autocracy. These divisions were later exploited by the colonial state to shape and comprehend Malagasy identities and to facilitate political control. In the process, concepts of identity have been forged in such a way that ethnic status has become far more important to outsiders than it is to those who are said to comprise the ethnic groups while, as in mainland Africa, ethnicity has come to be a means by which people can negotiate their identities in order to situate themselves politically and socially.

Archer (1978) points out that as in other countries considered "primitive," tribalism is invoked as the fundamental conflict hindering economic and political development in Madagascar. He argues that on the contrary, despite differences in certain customs, beliefs, and dialects, the Malagasy are primarily a homogeneous population whose differences throughout the history of unification in the 18th and 19th centuries, have predominately originated in economic and political, rather than ethnic, conflicts.

For example, French colonization facilitated the emergence of a wealthy Merina class, living primarily in Antananarivo but with close links to wealthy merchants and landowners throughout the island. Their accumulation of wealth had been possible because they had previously benefitted from Protestant educations and influential status in administrative posts during the Merina monarchy (Bloch 1986:31-32). At the same time, descendants of slaves and other free people among the Merina emerged as an impoverished, landless class who had more in common with their rural counterparts than they did with other Merina. The French promoted sufficient propaganda, however, to create the impression of religious and ethnic divisions characterizing internal conflicts between Merina and non-Merina, and Protestant and anti-Protestant factions, rather than the actual class divisions that prevail and which were only loosely related to Protestantism through its historical role in education and administration.

These class divisions, which separated people within regions, were obscured further as social divisions became characterized as geographical divisions; social conflict became perceived as being between people from the high plateaux and people from the coastal regions (e.g. Pryor 1990:202). Indeed, the geographical distribution of people has had significant bearing on how ethnicity has been perceived by early scholars (e.g. Linton 1939) as well as more contemporary writers describing the island (e.g. Stevens 1999). Madagascar was settled approximately 1500 to 2000 years ago by two groups: Indonesian seafarers who slowly migrated inland to settle in the high plateaux regions where malaria was less common, and Bantu seafarers who settled along the western coastal areas where they established trading communities (Kent 1970; Kottak 1980). As further population migrations dispersed throughout the island, lighter-skinned descendants of Indonesians, with straight hair and fine features, were among the first to receive the favorable attention of Europeans in their support of the Merina kingdom. As people were abducted into slavery from the coastal regions, it came to be that darker skinned people in the highlands were more likely to be descended from slaves, while lighter skinned people were more likely to be descended from slave holders.

But early ethnographic accounts pointed to endogamy to explain the history of how lighter and darker-skinned people became socially segregated, such as this summary by Ralph Linton (1939:251) in his discussion of "The Culture of Madagascar":

> The races are extremely diverse, great multiplicity of type being favored by endogamous group patterns. But certain main racial types are distinguishable with a fair degree of localization. In the plateau, the bulk of the population is mesocephalic, with light brown skin, long wavy hair, fairly heavy beard, and straight eyes.

Linton (1957:26,27) extended his argument further to presume a moral culpability of the darker phenotype, as he ignored the relationship of Madagascar's industrialization to disease distribution, by attributing the spread of malaria in pre-colonial Africa to Bantu descendants whom he charges virtually exterminated the seemingly superior race:

> In Madagascar, brown people of southeast Asiatic origin occupy the central plateau of the island where there were no anopheles mosquitoes until they were introduced by the building of a railroad from the coast. Completely surrounding this island of Asiatics was a belt of Negroid peoples who occupy all the fever infected coastal lowlands. One of the most interesting aspects of this situation was that the Negroid people all speak Malayo-Polynesian languages and have cultures which show a strong Asiatic tinge. There can be little doubt that they arrived on the island after the Malayo-Polynesians by a process of gradual infiltration rather than mass settlement. They presumably brought malaria with them from Africa, with the result that the Asiatic racial type was eliminated in all areas where there were fever carrying mosquitoes, although not before the Asiatics had transmitted much of their culture to the Negro immigrants.

The separation of Malagasy peoples according to their phenotype has been indiscriminately glossed as Merina and non-Merina populations, conferring an ethnic identity onto these "racial" categories. Campbell (1985) suggests that the concept of racial superiority of Merina over darker-skinned Malagasy was further facilitated by European evolutionists who argued that the lighter skin and skeletal physiology of the Merina suggested closer resemblance to European physiognomy and hence, greater intelligence.

This conflation of ethnicity with race is still deeply embedded in concepts of Malagasy society. For example, Huntington (1988:3,4) cites Michel (1957) as equating ethnic identification with race:

> The author of one study of the Bara cited the "fact" that Bara "skin is frankly black and impregnated with the strong odor characteristic of the Bantu" as evidence that the social and religious system of the Bara is essentially African.

More than thirty years later, Murphy (1985:10) writes:

> The exact origin of the Merina, the largest and most enterprising of Madagascar's eighteen main tribes, remains a mystery. Scholars offer contradictory explanations for their light brown skin, straight black hair and impeccable Polynesian features... The minority of Merina who do not look pure Polynesian tend to be tallish and rather dark with slightly wavy hair....

And finally, writing for the World Bank, Pryor (1990:202) offers this simple description of social differences:

> Ethnic frictions do exist, however, and have a strongly regional focus. In "high politics" the most important cleavage is between the peoples of the highlands (primarily Merina and Betsileo) and the rest of the island (the coastal peoples, or the *cotiers*) (see Spacensky 1970). *Aside from the racial differences between these two groups*, these cleavages are accentuated by a number of important economic and cultural factors [emphasis added].

Before showing more specifically how these social divisions have been represented by policy makers in respect to the environment and health and healing practices, I discuss how three such "ethnic" groups central to this regional study came to be constructed, namely, the Merina, Betsileo, and the Tanala.

Forging Ethnicities

In addition to the economic and land reforms instituted by Andrianampoinimerina, the early nineteenth century economic and political expansion of the new kingdom required that cultural belief systems be manipulated. *Ombiasa* [healers] and *mpanjaka* [village or lineage leaders] were used by the pre-colonial ruler to promote a world view in which certain classes of people were divinely privileged over others. Viewing their authority as precariously positioned in the changing social order, many cultural leaders promoted the new policies. Social cohesion loosened as respect for leadership gave way to fear of leadership. A Merina ethnicity emerged in which solidarity with the new royal leaders was pitted against 'the other,' non-Merina ethnicities (a strategy emulated by the French colonialists a century later [Andriambelomiadana 1992]).

There are no references to Merina as a social group prior to the nineteenth century; it is likely that a Merina ethnic identity did not emerge until the late eighteenth century (Larson 1996, 1992). Prior to that, inland communities shared common ideologies, cosmologies, rituals, principles of social organization and politics, but were not collectively identified (aside from derogatory references made of them as "dog-pigs" [Larson 1992:86]). It was not until 1792, when Andrianampoinimerina moved his kingdom to Antananarivo, that the terms Merina and Imerina (the place of the Merina), were geographically extended and gained popularity among the local people. This period, Larson (1992) suggests, was when social practices now associated with Merina traditions (such as irrigated rice agriculture and burial in "ancestral" tombs) emerged as explicit ethnic practices, distinguishing privileged groups from the subjugated groups of the expanding empire. Merina ethnic identity, he argues, was fashioned in part by a few ruling elite who sought to diffuse social discontent in the highlands (Larson 1992).

The forging of ethnicity was directly linked to the reorganization of land during the rise of the Merina monarchy. One of the most significant tactics Andrianampoinimerina employed to assure his success was to invent an ethnic tradition and social structure in which island groups would be distinct and identifiable (Larson 2000, 1992). Specifically, the king was interested in forging a social identity tied to the royal court:

> For his part, by striving to politically appropriate all highland Madagascar for himself, Andrianampoinimerina sought to generate a novel sense of highland political identity, one loyal to his kingdom-building project. As crosscutting royal and popular strategies for the transformation of political relationships confronted one another in highland Madagascar, they shifted identity politics to center stage and nurtured a new, complex, and locally textured political identity in highland Madagascar — being Merina (Larson 2000:162).

Toward his objective of forging a Merina ethnicity, the highland king popularized ancestral tombs and ancestral land (*tanindrazana*). The official demarcating of land holdings was very important to Andrianampoinime-rina's land policy, in order to prevent other rulers from attracting follow-ers, and to ensure the collection of taxes (Campbell 1985; Larson 1992). The new *hetra*, not necessarily ancestral to those to whom they were as-signed (having in most cases recently migrated as a result of warfare or to escape slavery), were recast as ancestral lands by Andrianampoinimerina. Anyone who did not support the "ancestral land" was to be publicly dri-ven away by the *fokonolona* and his *hetra* seized and given to others. The manipulating of this ancestral tradition continued through the nineteenth century, creating a new ethnic "Merina" identity that previously did not exist (Bloch 1986; Feeley-Harnik 1991; Larson 1992).[1]

Each *tanindrazana* and ancestral tomb would have its own relationship to the king, its own history, and its own set of rules and social order. This construction of ethnicity served to assure the loyalty of the *firenenena* (small-scale corporate descent groups organized around political leaders to designate the kingdom) to the king and provide a sense of safety and security to rural inhabitants.

Deepening Social Divisions and Castes

As Andrianampoinimerina initiated his land reorganization policies that were to later become state policies in the early nineteenth century, he linked them to social restructuring. The emergence of class divisions, clearly triggered long before with concepts of sovereignty and serfdom, were rapidly fixed in the new society. Landlessness or near landlessness, differ-ing access to resources, monetization of the economy, monopolization of the slave trade by an elite group of chiefs and kings, and the introduction of foreign-owned or -controlled industry, all served to dispossess the ma-jority of the population of the means of their production and to facilitate social divisions based on caste.

Andrianampoinimerina, while not establishing caste divisions himself, capitalized on them to give credence to his dominion.[2] To do so, however, it was first critical to justify to the public the necessity of slavery. One way

---

1. Imerina had been documented as a place name, but it was not until the early nine-teenth century that Merina is mentioned as an ethnic group (Larson 1992).

2. Campbell (1985) reports that it was King Andriamasinavalona (1675-1710) who laid the foundation for a caste-based society by restricting such castes to a specific area of Imerina and imposing compulsory state service (the irrigation of rice fields). Following his death, civil wars fragmented the region until Andrianampoinimerina rose in power and reinstituted Andriamasinavalona's techniques.

Andrianampoinimerina succeeded in this effort was by exploiting the authority of the *ombiasa* [shaman, or divination specialist and healer], by propagating the myth that the deity Zanahary had fixed the destiny of each person, and that people were not equal in the eyes of Zanahary, who had created some with more elevated destinies than others (Beaujard 1983:388). It is possible that the *mpanjaka* [village chief or one who governs], viewing their authority as precarious in the new social order, used their divination skills to contribute to the perpetuation of this myth, in order that their political strength be viewed as divinely determined (Beaujard 1983).

Four broad social divisions were then advanced. These were the *andriana*[3] (nobles by birthright), *hova*[4] (free people), *mainty* (emancipated slaves[5], including descendants of *hova* who had been reduced to slavery), and *andevo* (slaves) (Dubois 1938). Slaves were forbidden from owning land, thereby rendering them dependant on *hova* or *andriana*.

Campbell (1985) suggests that the Merina social structure resembles not so much a class system, in which economic mobility is theoretically possible, as it does a caste system.[6] In this caste system, the *hova* were elevated in status only as the *andevo* were absorbed through forced labor and slavery. Each new Merina social group, as in India, was absorbed as a new caste, according to Campbell. Moreover, to maintain such a caste system, it was necessary to enforce rules of endogamy, which was done by legislating family law and restricting each caste to a specific territory from which they could not move without royal consent (Campbell 1985). The concentration of caste, Campbell notes, provided a concentration of labor resources. Therefore, by concentrating *hova* and *andevo* castes in the eastern forested regions, their labor could be appropriated to exploit the forest resources.

Bloch (1989), however, suggests that ethnographers have mistakenly emphasized concepts of caste divisions to understand Malagasy social dif-

---

3. The *andriana* are frequently invoked as a "traditional" class of royalty. Dubois (1938) however, argued that the formation of the *andriana* caste was defined by Ralambo (who ruled from 1615-1640), and is therefore, of relatively recent social innovation.

4. Dubois (1938) points out that the term "*hova*" is problematic, because among the Betsileo the term refers exclusively to descendants of chiefs and the privileged class. Among the Imerina, however, the term refers to all free people and means "second class."

5. In some cases, a slave was able to work or buy his or her freedom, while in other cases, slave status was permanent.

6. Linton (1933) had also noted the resemblance to a caste system, but pointed out that such a type of social organization was not uniform throughout the island, and even within the limited territory of the Tanala, there were differences. For example, the southern Ikongo were organized more like a caste system, than were the northern Menabe.

ferences, and in so doing, have equated these social divisions with linguistic categories. Instead, although Bloch recognizes similarities to the Indian caste system, he argues that social separation among highland Malagasy during the Merina empire was not clearly marked among *andriana*, *hova*, and *andevo*. Within each rank there existed several gradations of social status. Although a slim minority of those identified as *andriana* ruled the majority, not all *andriana* could be classified as rulers, and among the other categories, there remained many differences in terms of social power. Bloch (1989) finds that the more salient social divisions are not the categories of *andriana*, *hova* and *andevo*, but are more clearly understood in terms of what he calls *demes*, or descent groups, organized around one or more linked rice valleys (Bloch 1989:51).

> This is where the division in terms of power exists: between some members of a *deme* and the rest, consisting of other members of their *deme* together with the members of all other *demes* (Bloch 1989:62).

Bloch goes on to indicate that all members of the same *deme* have the same rank, but may have very different levels of political power. This point is significant, because it underscores the ways in which contemporary social divisions cannot be understood merely in terms of a caste system in which members are undifferentiated, but points instead to the ways in which social differences within castes are salient to contemporary power relations.

Emergence of Betsileo and Tanala Ethnicities

The Betsileo were an administrative construction of the Merina autocracy (Kottak 1971a). The area which is now regarded as Betsileo territory was first populated around 1700. Andrianampoinimerina, seeking to control the mass populace and the fertile lands, organized the island into six administrative divisions. This administrative reorganization began as small surveillance posts around which provinces were formed (Kottak 1971a). Kottak (1971a:136) stressed this point in his ethnography of the Betsileo.

> Many of the ethnic units enumerated in the Malagasy census originated as labels for provincial and territorial divisions of the Merina state. Employed also by the French, they were reinforced, and today they ascribe ethnic status for life.

In the case of the Betsileo and Bara, Kottak (1971a) indicated that the Merina constructed their ethnicity by demarcating an administrative line between two provinces. One, which came to be known as Betsileo, had its capital at Fianarantsoa, and the other, to be designated as Bara, had its capital at Ihosy, in the north. These administrative divisions were gradually regarded as ethnic distinctions.

The administrative divisions of the Betsileo and the Merina were further reinforced by the colonial administration. Allen (1995:124) points to this process of reifying ethnicity:

> The extent of "tribalism" in Malagasy politics has often been exaggerated to disguise other animosities of political elites, social classes, or religion. It is nonetheless true that political and social privileges originating in the nineteenth-century internal colonialism of the Merina have engendered considerable resentment among other Malagasy. Chaigneau identifies the role of the French colonial administration in perpetuating the conflict: "The colonial government bequeathed a practice of exploiting the bitterness emergent from situations of domination, while building an anthropological and ethnological literature aiming at 'scientific' justification of this opposition. This was the product of an analysis which proved effective and convenient in controlling the country but which scarcely considered sociological realities."

One strategy toward this end was French colonial Governor Gallieni's *politique des races*. Governor Gallieni was the first colonial governor to control Madagascar, taking control with the occupation of Madagascar in 1895, and colonial annexation in 1896.

Allen suggests that the *politique des races* was a colonial effort to institute a quasi-affirmative action campaign in which coastal groups were targeted for educational and economic opportunities to facilitate social parity with the Merina (which the colonial government sought to disempower). In the end, however, the *politique des races* turned out to be an ineffective policy because, as Allen argues, the better-educated high-plateau "Merina" proved to be the more suitable job applicants for colonial administration, and colonial resources were too limited to implement the policies of the *politiques des races*. Thus, during the colonial period social disparity intensified between Merina and non-Merina, rather than lessened.

Whereas ethnic groups in Madagascar, as elsewhere, have been essentially political constructs, Kottak (1971a:136fn) notes that

> There have been exceptions in which ethnic designation is determined by environment rather than by political order. The Tanala inhabit the rainforest between the highlands and the east coast. The term Tanala means "people of the forest." Any-

one who lives in the forest and practices a Tanala horticultural economy is a Tanala. The common cultural adaptation confers a certain ethnic unity here.

Thus, Kottak makes two important points relevant to the ethnicity of the Betsileo and the Tanala. First, he suggests that the Betsileo, like most other of the eighteen "designated ethnic units" of the Malagasy population, are fairly recent administrative constructions, rather than self-distinguished sub-cultures of the greater Malagasy "culture." Second, he points out that the Tanala are not an administrative division, but are instead forest residents identified by the way they live within their environment. This conception of the Tanala as being defined by the way they live is similar to how Astuti has represented the concept of ethnicity among the Vezo. Astuti (1995) has shown how the Vezo, people of the west coast of Madagascar whose economic subsistence is based on fishing, are presumed to be an ethnic group based on descent, yet viewed from the perspective of the people themselves, Vezo is a performative category in which people become Vezo by living as Vezo.

> ... Vezo become what they are through what they do; both identity and difference result from activities that people perform in the present rather than from a common or distinct origin they acquired at some point in the past (Astuti 1995:465).

Her concept of "becoming" Vezo parallels Kottak's (1971b) view that anyone can become "Tanala," by practicing the economic strategies of the forest environment. The Tanala and the Betsileo, while treated as two different "ethnic groups," are, Kottak points out, two very different categories of people — one a political category of highland people administratively created by the nineteenth century Merina state, the other a geographical category of people who live within a certain environment and therefore practice certain economic strategies for effectively living within their environment — most notably, swidden agriculture.

These classifications are not absolute, however. Bloch (1995) has suggested that among the Zafimaniry of eastern Madagascar, who live in an environment which is not conducive to swidden rice agriculture, the practice of irrigated rice agriculture has been closely associated with their Betsileo neighbors. As the increasing loss of forest cover makes it more difficult for the Zafimaniry to practice swidden production of maize, beans and taro, they have begun changing their agricultural practices to include irrigated rice agriculture. As their land becomes cleared and suitable for irrigated rice production, and as they adopt the practice of irrigated farming, they say that they become "Betsileo." Thus, the administrative division of the Betsileo does have a performative aspect, but it is not the fixed ethnic label assumed by some; rather, because it is performative, it is a permeable category.

Ethnic identity can and does change, but in different ways for different people. In the Ranomafana region, one does not become Betsileo by practicing irrigated rice farming. Instead, because irrigated rice farming is practiced alongside swidden rice production, "Betsileo" become "Tanala," a concept that is less conceived of as an ethnic one, as it is a way of living. The difference between the "Zafimaniry" views of Betsileo as a performative category, and "Tanala" views of Betsileo as a category of descent, does not, in my view, suggest a contradiction as much as an affirmation that ethnic identity is permeable, with differing meanings for differing groups. To clarify this point, I draw on how Betsileo and Tanala were presented by Kottak (1971b), because it is his presentations of Tanala and Betsileo ethnicity that most contributed to how ethnicity was perceived by those park administrators I encountered who expressed familiarity with the local ethnography.

Building on Harris (1979), Kottak proposes a model of cultural adaptive types, rather than "ethnic" groups, to understand how different groups of people use the land in which they live. In so doing, he treats "Tanala" as swidden agriculturalists living in the forest, and "Betsileo" and "Merina" as irrigation agriculturalists living in the central highlands. He clearly illuminates the fallacy of regarding the Merina administrative divisions of the population as credible cultural boundaries, but uses the names of these groups to help identify people living within different environments. Thus, he groups "Merina" and "Betsileo" together as irrigation agriculturalists of the central highlands, as he does the "Tanala" and the "Betsimisaraka" (living in the central coastal forests northeast of the Ranomafana region) as swidden agriculturalists of the eastern escarpment. The analytical boundaries separating groups of people are, in this model, economic boundaries rather than ethnic ones; the economic strategies people practice are thereby made fundamental to understandings of social structure. Conceptualizing cultural identity, then, requires as much attention to economic relations as to ethnicity.

Kottak's conceptualization of adaptive types echoes Linton's argument that the social distinction separating Betsileo from Tanala does not arise from descent, but instead from economic practices:

> Tanala and Betsileo cultures were identical in the main. The differences are traceable to the change in productive methods from dry to wet rice cultivation. This is proven by several circumstances: The traditions in Betsileo indicate an old culture very like Tanala; the institutions of both indicate a common source, and many of them are still identical; the changes in

Tanala were gradual, and were well on the way to becoming identical with Betsileo when the French took over; and finally some of the Tanala tribes took over the wet rice method and abandoned it because of the serious incompatibilities it created in the social structure. The spread of wet rice cultivation cannot be attributed solely to diffusion; wet rice culture was endemic in Tanala and coincident with dry rice. Its spread was favored largely by exhaustion of the dry method. Hence in examining the changes secondary to this main innovation, we need not depend exclusively on diffusion for an explanation (Linton 1939:290).

The history of wet-rice and swidden rice agriculture is therefore more clearly understood by examining the historical and social factors shaping land use, rather than summarizing Betsileo and Tanala "cultures" as a series of unrelated traits, and presuming the practice of *tavy* to be embedded in such an ambiguously defined cultural belief system.

Honoring Tradition: "Cultural Sensitivity" and the RNPP

As discussed in the Introduction, fundamental to the Ranomafana National Park Project's conceptualization of the social and environmental relationships shaping the loss of species biodiversity in the Ranomafana region, was the view that *tavy* rice production threatened lemur survival by destroying the primates' forest habitat. The project therefore identified swidden agriculture, or *tavy*, as the greatest ecological threat to the region's biodiversity (RNPP 1994). The most important economic and social strategy of the RNPP administration was to encourage the shift from swidden rice agriculture (*tavy*) to irrigated rice agriculture (*tanim-bary*), a strategy which failed for the colonial administration. To compensate the residents for loss of the forest lands, the Project promised improved health care, sanitation, contraception, education and revenues from the National Park.

To gain understanding of the perceptions and needs of the local villagers, members of the RNPP and representatives of the Department of Water and Forest visited all the villages surrounding the proposed national park. This survey took seven six-day trips on foot over steep terrain.

The average village housed 300 individuals who lived in about thirty adobe mud huts with thatched rooms. We met with the village elders first, then had a general meeting with the population of each village. The elders discussed the need for schools, health clinics, and technical assistance with agriculture. As we listened, the scope of the project increased. For long-term success in protecting any habitat we need to be realistic and begin with incorporating the needs of the people who live adjacent to the protected area from the beginning (Wright 1992:28).

Nonetheless, rewards were not forthcoming, a failure that the national and international institutions supporting the project noted early on:

The project has raised high expectations among the local villagers that cannot be met. And unfortunately, pilot projects do not address this issue. The equitable distribution of benefits to villagers in compensation for the loss of resources of the park needs to be given highest priority (DEF/USAID/ANGAP Debriefing, 7/12/93, General Observations).

That the project promised social benefits in exchange for rights to forest land is clear. What is less clear is how residents were selected to receive these benefits. As with many development projects, those villages located closest to the road—and therefore more visible to consultants, reporters and tourists—received more benefits.[7]

Ambatolahy is a village five miles from Ranomafana, just off the n[?] road. It is near the entrance to the park in what scientists call high humid cloud forest. All seven of the park guides [the Principle Investigator of the RNPP] has hired to lead tourists into the park come from this town (Bohlen 1993:27)....During our return trip she stops at a village at the park trailhead to present a toilet seat she had brought from the United States for installation in its privy. (Will other villages be envious? Will she have to order twenty-five more?) At her suggestion this village has also built a thatched-roofed snack bar. Here the villagers sell soft drinks to thirsty hikers with an appealing shyness bordering on diffidence. A noncash economy is reaping its first monetary payment from the park; a service industry is being born though no one quite realizes it (Bohlen 1993:36).

Paul Hanson, an ethnographer who conducted fieldwork in the Ranomafana region from 1992-1994, has also shown how the village of Ambodiaviavy received hurricane relief aid from the park, as well as other

---

7. See Chambers (1983) and Hancock (1989) on beneficiaries of development projects.

benefits (Hanson 1997), while the centrally located town of Ranomafana was rewarded with numerous construction projects and local businesses are provided with periodic coats of whitewash.

But how those villages off the road have been selected for project benefits, particularly for health care, is related more to perceived agricultural practices and ethnic identity than it is to putting on a good show. In determining how social benefits would be distributed, the project focused on what it considered to be the social factors contributing to the environmental destruction in the area. More specifically, the project attempted to address local social factors contributing to the practice of *tavy*. While on the surface, such an objective suggests concern for incorporating cultural beliefs and behaviors into policy, the ways in which social factors were determined to be salient reflected the administrative perspective that local practices were the *cause* of environmental degradation. For example, the relationship between urban resource use and environmental change, the historical context of farming in the Ranomafana region, and the social changes associated with structural adjustment and the influx of outsiders associated with the RNPP itself, were not included in this focus of social factors contributing to the practice of *tavy*.

What the administration did do, however, was to identify two "ethnic groups" in the region—the Tanala, and the Betsileo, representing the early settlers and the later immigrants, respectively.

> Two ethnic groups live within the buffer zone: the Betsileo people of the Western highlands and the Tanala people who mainly live in lower elevations in the central and eastern regions of the park. There is much intermingling between the two groups (RNPP 1994:4).

According to project documents, the agricultural practices of the residents are distinguished by ethnicity.

> Two basic forms of subsistence agriculture are practiced by farmers in the peripheral zone...The Tanala people traditionally practice slash and burn agriculture or "tavy."...The use of tavy has had a considerable negative environmental impact in the eastern cloud forest and lowlands. Since 1960 it is estimated that 50% of the existing forests have been cut, mainly for tavy...The Betsileo people traditionally cultivate paddy rice in relatively flat land around rivers and streams (RNPP 1994:5).

While "the Betsileo people" are regarded as traditional paddy rice cultivators, *tavy* is viewed as the "tradition" of the Tanala (RNPP 1994:16).

The advantages of tavy agriculture are that it often yields more than paddy rice, especially in the first year, it is easier to cultivate, local people can't afford chemical fertilizer necessary for paddy rice, multiple crops can be planted in tavy fields, fewer tools are needed for tavy, guarding the fields is not necessary and cattle can graze on the residue. One important aspect of this agricultural system is cultural in that the Tanala people have traditionally practiced tavy (RNPP 1994:16).

The project thus describes the economic and pragmatic reasons why *tavy* is practiced, but concludes that an important aspect of why it is practiced is cultural "in that the Tanala people have traditionally practiced *tavy*" (RNPP 1994:16). The reasons why people practice a certain farming strategy is thus reduced to a timeless, non-rational notion of "tradition." In other words, even though the system makes sense economically, it is practiced by the "Tanala" for "cultural" reasons, because it is their "tradition."

They are further said to be inexperienced with irrigated rice farming, and must depend upon "Betsileo" labor to do it for them.

Most Tanala villagers, and even some Betsileo villagers in the central section of the park, are not skilled at working on rice paddies. Having inhabited the region for more than a century and having depended mainly on tavy agriculture, they have lost much of the necessary knowledge, if indeed they ever had it at all. For the last five to six decades, or longer in some cases, many Tanala households have used migrant Betsileo laborers from the High Plateau to work their rice paddies. Peters (1993:190) reports that in one Tanala village, residents "may even leave the rice paddies idle if they do not have enough money to employ the Betsileo to complete all the paddies" (Ferraro and Rakotondrajaona 1992).

The "Tanala" are further characterized by a social organization in which power is vested in the *mpanjaka* [village or lineage leaders], and women have relatively little power in comparison to the "Betsileo" (Ferraro 1994). It is alleged that due to their "tradition" and their "culture," they have been resistant to the project strategies to increase irrigated rice fields. As such, "Tanala" are conceptualized as posing the greatest social threat to the "ecosystem."

RNPP development activities during Phase II will rely on a prioritized approach to address threats identified in the three target areas: 1) non-sustainable, consumptive utilization of forest products 2) sustainable, consumptive utilization of forest products and 3) sustainable, non-consumptive utilization of the forest. *These activities will be tailored to take into account ethnic variations of resource use* and economic stratification patterns within peripheral zone communities (RNPP 1994:24, emphasis added).

The "Betsileo," in contrast are viewed by the project as being more amenable to irrigated rice farming, more experienced with agricultural innovations, and more educated. Their social structure is distinguished from the "Tanala," in that power is represented as more "democratic," with village elders and women having authority in decision-making regarding resource use. Moreover, like the supposed "Tanala," the social structure and agricultural practices of the "Betsileo" are said to be rooted in their "traditions" and their "culture" (RNPP 1994:5).

This dichotomizing of village residents by their ethnicity provides a circular reasoning by which the project classifies people. If they practice irrigated rice farming, they are Betsileo; if they are Betsileo, they practice irrigated rice farming. If they are *tavy* farmers, they are "Tanala," if they are "Tanala," they are *tavy* farmers. Not only does this view presume that farmers practice a single agricultural strategy, which is not the case, this view also treats the fact that the northern, southern, and central regions are flatter, with more land conducive to wet-rice agriculture, as coincident to ethnicity. The eastern "Tanala" region is much more topographically constrained—very little land is suitable to irrigated rice farming, yet the practice of swidden farming is regarded by the project as "ancestral tradition," borne of this topography perhaps, but, over time, has become so firmly fixed in the "Tanala" mind as the way of the ancestors that they are incapable of adopting new farming practices unless they have no other choice.

This ethnic stereotyping has impeded both groups from receiving development assistance. Prior to the project, UNICEF provided assistance to the Malagasy government to target those they identified as Betsileo for receiving credit to buy fertilizers and other agricultural inputs, because they were allegedly more responsive to increasing wet-rice production. Subsequently, presuming that it is the "Tanala" who need the most "*sensibilization*," the project targeted those they identified as "Tanala"—based on the extent to which they practice tavy—to receive the benefits of agricultural extension. Working to incorporate the supposed "Tanala culture" into its scheme, the project both aimed to obliterate *tavy*, while catering to the perceived traditions of a "Tanala" ethnic identity. At the same time, they embraced a neo-colonial policy of indirect rule, in which agricultural change was facilitated by working within the village social structures in the name of "participation."

The programs will attempt to work through local power structures to address the cultural aspect of tavy as well as through educational and technical programs that look at the production levels of the crops and alternatives.....Targeted groups of residents will be those who have historically been involved in cutting virgin forest lands. These people include young or poor households who have not inherited land, migrants who have no designated land and older people who contend that use of the forest is their right. Programs will be concentrated mainly in villages on the eastern side of the park where population densities are the greatest and tavy is utilized extensively. The western region of the park and the areas of the high plateau, which are mainly inhabited by Betsileo, have no tavy tradition and land that is more conducive to paddy rice. These areas will be excluded from the programs unless individual villages are identified as posing a significant threat (RNPP 1994:22).

Moreover, Hanson (1993) suggests that the ways in which Project planners have stereotyped local populations in terms of ethnicity may have profound effects in the manipulation of cultural rituals to legitimate claims to land, and might lead to other recontextualizations of folklore and ritual. He, too, points to the ways in which ethnic stereotypes have been reproduced by the project and divorced from political and historical context, drawing attention to the ways in which such stereotypes correspond to degrees of social contact:

> In planning many of these projects, Park researchers have delimited a population who they believe pose the most immediate threat to the area's forests. Park development, sociological, and health team discourses, in representing the needs of this population, have reproduced some long-standing ethnic stereotypes. The Betsileo, located to the north and west of the protected area, have an extensive history of contact with the more "developed" Merina and French populations in the highlands. Because of this association, the Betsileo are said to be hard working farmers, competent with wet rice agriculture and open to Park innovation. It is only poverty, population growth and landlessness that has forced these populations into *tavy*. The Tanala, on the other hand, remained relatively isolated from highland influences (Hanson 1993:338).

Hanson further shows how the project draws on stereotypes of local political structures, which they associate with ethnic categories, to explain agricultural practices.

> According to Ranomafana National Park socio-economic discourses, the Tanala *mpanjaka* (governors), unlike the more

democratically-oriented Betsileo leaders, wield complete control over the distribution of resources. The *mpanjaka's* monopoly over the village's wet rice fields forces younger farmers and more recent immigrants into *tavy* production. Because the *mpanjaka* are concerned with maintaining such privileged positions, Tanala traditional authority is seen as a major obstacle to Park "development" projects (Peters 1992:234-237; Samisoa 1992:134-135; Ranomafana National Park staff, personal communications) (Hanson 1993:339).

Contrary to the *mpanjaka* of Ranotsara controlling the irrigated rice fields and undermining democratic processes, it is instead those who have most benefitted from the project itself who control the most land in Ranotsara. I will return to some of the issues Hanson raises in subsequent chapters, but at this point it is important to emphasize that by gaining control of land and labor, power has become concentrated among a few families in the village; while most people, including indigenous leaders and elders, have lost both real and, to a lesser extent, symbolic power. These changing power relations have contributed to the local environmental crisis in Ranotsara, a process common to post-colonial societies (Bryant and Bailey 1997). Nonetheless, those who do hold power locally, remain relatively powerless in their community in comparison to the power wielded by national and international outsiders who control the use of the surrounding forests, health and agricultural policies, and the national economy. By focusing on ethnicity as the defining feature by which to understand the complex relationships between environmental change and local culture, those who live beyond the boundaries of the forests and yet who control environmental and economic policies of the forests, remain shielded from deeper understandings of how differing levels of power influence human and environmental relations.

Rather than focusing on ethnicity to understand processes of deforestation, a more fruitful line of inquiry focuses on the relationship between agricultural practices and social structures in order to illuminate contemporary power structures affecting environmental change. In an article well-known to scholars of Madagascar, and which can be found on the shelves of the RNPP library, Oxby (1985) has argued that historical changes, not "traditional" reverence for the *mpanjaka*, have shaped power structures in Malagasy farming communities.

The transformation of land use from forest to farm is gradual: the ancestors of the irrigated-rice cultivators of the central plateau area of Madagascar were hill rice cultivators several centuries ago, when the area was covered by forest. Gradually, as the forest was destroyed, they turned to irrigated agriculture. In some cases, people were pushed back into the forest as a result of wars and reverted to hill rice cultivation (Bloch 1975).

Instructive also is the social transformation, from a sparse population of forest dwellers living in semi-permanent settlements whose social organization is relatively egalitarian, to a village-based society characterized by higher population densities and a more hierarchical social structure. These parallel changes in land use and society are important in understanding the farmers' choice of agricultural strategy (Oxby 1985:43).

If, then, rice cultivation is a result of historical circumstances, how is it that people's histories have been replaced with their ethnicities? As Hanson (1997) argues, stereotypes, rather than empirical research, shape discourse on populations in the Ranomafana region. He ties contemporary stereotypes to colonial representations of the Tanala and Betsileo.

> These colonial understandings of the Tanala as lazy and unconcerned with the future of the forests constitute the historical precedents for RNPP attitudes toward the Tanala of the Ranomafana region. Most RNPP socioeconomic studies distinguish between the Betsileo living to the west and north of the RNP, and the Tanala, occupying the areas south and east of the Park. "The Tanala," we are told, "traditionally practice tavy...cultivation," whereas the Betsileo, who in the past planted rice in the valley fields, "have now begun practicing tavy since arriving in the region, due in part to the topographical constraints" (Ferraro & Rakotondrajaona 1992:6). In Madagascar, tavy and wet-rice cultivation occasion very different responses from observers. Ferraro and Rakotondrajaona argue that "many Malagasy and foreign people who come to Ranomafana from other areas comment that the locals in this region, especially the Tanala, are lazy. They say that the Tanala prefer tavy because it is easier; that they don't work very hard on their rice paddies, preferring to pay migrant Betsileo to work on them. These observations are partly true" (ibid:10). As the historical sketches I presented above make clear, these observations are absurd. However, such stereotypes are the norm in the RNPP (Hanson 1997:103).

As Hanson (1993:338-339) further indicates, the discourses of ethnicity employed by the RNPP neglect informed understandings of how the Betsileo and Tanala ethnic distinctions have evolved. In addition, I contend that they also reflect weak understandings of the broader academic scholarship on ethnicity and culture.

Young (1986) distinguishes two primary models of ethnicity: the instrumentalist model, which treats ethnicity as a political concept based on competition and self-interest, and the primordial model, which treats ethnicity as a cultural phenomenon, based on historical tradition.

In discussing Tanala and Betsileo ethnicity, D. Peters (1994b), employs an instrumentalist model in an effort to make the project more egalitarian. Using stereotypes of the "Tanala" as *tavy* farmers who have no knowledge of irrigated rice agriculture and are less "developed" than the "Betsileo," she aims to increase "Tanala" participation in the project and bring them closer to "Betsileo" standards of living.

> These data show that the exclusion of the resident peoples from the natural resources within the park boundary means disruption of household economy, more time allocated to working, and loss of natural resources for a variety of purposes. The most serious impact perhaps rests in the impact on cultural identity, if the project is to succeed in banning *tavy*. The data also suggest that impacts on the Tanala and the remote villages will likely be stronger than on the Betsileo because the life of the Tanala and the remote villages is more connected to converting and exploiting the natural resources.... Because the Betsileo in general own more paddy fields, it is likely that they may benefit more from introduced technologies (e.g., water management and organic and chemical fertilizer application) than the Tanala; the households that are fortunate to own more paddies are likely to benefit more (D. Peters 1994b:9).

Peters' image of "Tanala" as *tavy* farmers and "Betsileo" as irrigated rice farmers is the one most often cited in project documents; unfortunately, it was her *image* of ethnicity that the project incorporated, not her aim. Peters' main point is that those most disenfranchised and impoverished should become principle beneficiaries of any development aid, including health aid. A class or caste analysis which is divorced from ethnicity more accurately represents the local populations, thereby illuminating her call for a more egalitarian project. The project, however, appears to have closed its ears to her main point, brandishing only the stereotypical images she employed in its effort to address the cultural needs of the population.

Hanson, conversely, employs the "primordial" model Young identifies, in his efforts to situate *tavy* in history and record "Tanala" "consciousness." His efforts to historicize the "Tanala" are aimed at contextualizing contemporary views and practices as transformative and reasoned, rather than the ageless "tradition" and irrationality of *tavy* portrayed by the Ranomafana National Park Project.

> For the Tanala, the economic and cultural aspects of *tavy* cannot be separated. Rather than being a non-sustainable means

to meet basic needs as the RNPP argues, *tavy* represents a historical response to such forces as slavery, forced labor, taxation, forced export agricultural production, and pre-colonial and colonial forest policies. The most significant regionalization process for the Tanala in recent memory is the creation of the Ranomafana National Park and the establishment of the RNPP (Hanson 1997:83).

Yet both these models of ethnic groups presume economic and social homogeneity (Banks 1996:13), and therefore make understanding of culture fairly simple, reducible to a pat set of beliefs, traditions, and taboos.

Barth (1969) suggested that it is the boundaries between groups which are salient to ethnicity, not the cultural content they enclose. He rejected the idea that ethnic identity is a collection of traits, in favor of understanding those traits that the actors themselves consider significant. How one identifies him or herself, as compared to others, illuminates the boundaries that are salient to the social groups themselves—not to outsiders. Larson (1992; 1996), however, challenges Barth's noted concept of ethnicity, by suggesting that boundaries cannot pre-exist the content which they allegedly enclose. Larson's approach to content is directed toward an understanding of the multiple roles and relationships within a social group from which common identities are forged.

> By shifting our sight from inter-ethnic relationships at the border to intra-ethnic transactions at the center, the active roles of those consistently under-represented in traditional narratives emerges with greater clarity. In this light the process of ethnogenesis becomes a complex one in which contending and multiple purposes, intentions, interests and interpretations might be discerned. Ethnic groups no longer appear as monolithic blocks of identity confronting one another but as arenas where a common identity is both forged and debated (Larson 1992:5).

In his study of Merina ethnicity, Larson examines how the Merina themselves constructed a pre-colonial ethnicity in their interactions with the dominant economic forces of the late eighteenth century. His model for ethnogenesis can also be applied to understandings of Tanala ethnic identity in contemporary southeastern Madagascar. One can better understand Tanala culture by examining the competing and communal interests and identities among forest farmers who now socially identify themselves as practicing a "Tanala" lifestyle, but trace their ancestry to "Betsileo," rather than by compiling inventories of cultural traits.

Moreover, by linking its agricultural and environmental objectives to misconceived perceptions of local ethnic identities, the Ranomafana National Park Project fostered ambivalence among residents who redefined ethnic identities in order to either benefit from project assistance (as "Tanala") or to "rise" in status (as "Betsileo") while simultaneously revising their own or others' ancestry to justify increasing economic inequalities as inherent in one's caste.

In the following chapter I detail the history of two lineages in the village of Ranotsara, and describe how contemporary social life is positioned around these lineages. I contrast this representation of social organization to that which is portrayed by the Ranomafana National Park Project. I conclude by discussing how the project's conception of social organization has shaped the health care it has provided to residents and understandings of health and sickness. I suggest that these health services and perceptions replicate efforts by the colonial state to control populations and disregard the ramifications of policies to restructure the land and people of the island's forests.

Chapter 6

Dividing That Which Cannot Be Divided: Ancestry and Ethnicity in Ranotsara

As Erikson (1993:12) notes, "Only in so far as cultural differences are perceived as being important, and are made socially relevant, do social relationships have an ethnic element." The Ranomafana National Park Project regards agricultural practices as important and has focused on ethnicity as the divisive trait separating farmers. In this view, farming practices— ethnically distinguished—are regarded as relevant to conservation. But I found that the residents themselves value ancestry, its associated caste, and access to material resources as more salient social divisions. In the village of Ranotsara these internal social differences supercede the boundaries of ethnicity, and form the core of social identity. The residents of Ranotsara, most of whom identify themselves as descended from "Betsileo" but living as "Tanala", are united through their relationships to land and labor, while at the same time they are not so much divided by ethnicity as they are by both ancestry and economic differences.

Covell has discussed how ethnic identification in Madagascar has come to be embraced by Malagasy in efforts to access social benefits.

> Another organizing principle of Malagasy society and politics is that provided by the non-class solidarity ties of ethnicity, extended family, and locality. These lines of division are not unrelated to economic differences, and, indeed, much of the social and political importance of these groups comes from the use made of them as bases for individual and group protection and advancement. To a degree this cohesion rests on the belief that "in unity there is strength," but the groups also form useful bases for the phenomenon Schatzberg refers to as social closure. This is "the process by which social collectivities seek to maximize rewards by restricting access to a limited number of eligibles. This entails the singling out of certain identifiable social or physical attributes as the justificatory basis of exclusion" (1980, p.28). Similarly, Bates argues that the persistence of eth-

123

nic groups does not rest on the attachment of their members to 'traditional' values, but that "Ethnic groups persist largely because of their capacity to extract goods and services from the modern sector" (1974, p. 471) Covell (1987:81) .

Covell's argument that ethnicity persists in Madagascar because it enables certain groups of people to access resources, while excluding others from these resources, is a phenomenon witnessed in the Ranomafana region, where one's declared ethnic affiliation influenced access to resources associated with the modern sector promoted by the project. While residents themselves showed relatively little concern for ethnicity as compared to lineage, ethnicity remained the prevailing social distinction made by outsiders, particularly the Ranomafana National Park Project, as it set policy and negotiated access to economic resources and medicines.

In this chapter I discuss the founding of Ranotsara, the village in the southeastern forests of Madagascar in which I lived. From this founding two distinct lineages emerged. Descendants from these lineages comprise the present village population, and in my view, it is tensions between the lineages, rather than between ethnic affiliations, which explain current land management practices, economic status, and "cultural" behaviors and beliefs regarding health and healing. As members of the different lineages gained or lost prestige and power with the social changes of the twentieth century, conflicting histories of the lineages unfolded. At the same time, the shared history of resistance to outside control over local resources and livelihoods has contributed to social alliances that transcend community differences. These alliances are particularly acute in terms of how residents perceive conservation policies and their association with health resources. As the history of class and caste in Ranotsara is told, a simultaneous history is told of how a national park entered into the lives and bodies of the residents of this small village. In so doing, ethnicity became reified as the fundamental boundary separating farmers and households, and was used to explain spiraling sickness and death amidst what has been presented as a wonderland of natural medicines and a biodiversity of planetary bounty.

The Founding of a "Tanala" Village

Time is not marked by clocks or calendars in Ranotsara, at least not with a rigid adherence (plastic digital watches having made their appearance). According to the villagers, people often live to be a hundred years old, a hundred and twenty, a hundred and fifty, or more. A year past might be a year past, as a Westerner would mark it, but it might also be six months past or two years past. Time is instead marked by the seasons and the crops, and people are so busy living their lives according to the seasons and the crops, that they really haven't much time to mark the time. The past is *taloha* (in the past). And so it is difficult to know exactly when the village was founded, but it was agreed that it was founded sometime around the time of the French occupation, which began in 1895, when Madagascar became a protectorate of France (and a colony the following year).

According to village elders, Ranotsara was founded by two men, Rabiby, from the village of Ambatofady near Antananarivo, and Ramanjato, from the southwestern village of Analamena. Rabiby was of the Zafinaraina lineage and Ramanjato of the Zafindraraoto lineage. These two men established the village just under cliffs on a hill north of the current village, and named it Betsizaraina ("vast area that cannot be divided"). How close in time the men came is uncertain; what appears to be in agreement is that the *firenana* (lineage) of the Zafindraraoto lineage settled the area near Ranotsara first, which would make sense given that the Zafindraraoto lineage has a long history in the region. According to the elders of this lineage, and according to a project survey of the region (SAFAFI 1989), these founders were "Betsileo" *hova*, in other words, they were free men who came from the high plateaux. This status is important in understanding present land use patterns, and will be discussed subsequently.

Why they came is also unclear, but according to Faly, *mpanjaka* of the Zafindraraoto lineage in Ranotsara, his ancestor came from near the capital city of Antananarivo, migrating little by little before eventually settling in the present region with his wife. Faly emphasized that his ancestor was *hova*, but was not Merina. He wanted me to understand that the people of Ranotsara do not like the Merina. This point, and the way that he emphasized it, led me to believe that it was probable his ancestor migrated to avoid Merina (or Merina-influenced colonial) autocracy, which included the forced labor of *fanompoana* and taxation. At any rate, Faly was certain that his ancestor did not flee the highlands due to any wars. The other lineage that founded the village is the Zafinaraina lineage, which were said to be *andriana*, or noble caste.

According to elders from both lineages, the Zafindraraoto were adept at swidden horticulture. Because the Zafinaraina came from regions with land more suitable to pasturage and irrigated rice agriculture, they did not know how to farm the hills in this new terrain. As such, the Zafindraraoto taught them the technique of *tavy*, while the Zafinaraina showed the Zafindraraoto how to farm the limited flat lands at the base of the village.

The village moved, however, sometime during the early part of this century. It is not exactly clear whether the move was in association with colonial policies, but the explanation for the village's new name, Ranotsara, which means Good Water, is that at the old site, there was only one nearby river source, and the villagers used that for cooking, bathing, and drinking. They also used it to dump the old mats on which corpses lay decaying, and the old cloths they were wrapped in.

"Everytime someone died," Koto, an elder of the Zafinaraina lineage told me as we sat in his home eating boiled manioc, "there was a rush to the river so people could get their cooking and drinking water, and take a bath, before the *tsihy* [grass mats] were thrown in the river. So after the village moved, the *tsihy* were taken to sacred spots in the forest, and the river was clean."

Because the Zafindraraoto had settled the area before the Zafinaraina, they became the *tompontany*, or masters of the land. As such, to thank the Zafinaraina for teaching them the technique of wet-rice agriculture, according to Faly's younger brother, Tojo, the Zafindraraoto gave to the Zafinaraina some of the finest flat lands available in the new location, while they, too, took many flat lands but also retained some of the finest *tavy* fields, where their crops would be protected from cyclones, and where their skills were best perfected.

This account has been pieced together from discussions with several elderly informants from both lineages, and includes contradictory and ambiguous histories. But based on my knowledge of the history of the region, and based on their consistent reports that the Zafindraraoto gave the Zafinaraina land to thank them for teaching them farming techniques, I believe that this account is fairly accurate. It is particularly important in understanding that it is not the ethnicity of the two groups that determined which lands they farmed, nor in which manner, but it was lineage and experience.

The villagers were unanimous in asserting that both groups adapted the "Tanala" way of living, while maintaining ancestral connections to what became known as the "Betsileo."

The two lineages led to two types of *mpanjaka* [village chief, literally, "one who governs"]. These are the *mpitan-tranobe* [guardian of the big house] and the *mpitan-kazomanga* [guardian of the hazomanga—a sacred wood]. The *mpitan-tranobe* is the *mpanjaka* of the Zafinaraina lineage, which, as mentioned previously, was regarded as a long-established lineage of *andriana* (royal) descent. The *mpitan-tranobe* was also a *mpitan-kazomanga*, but because they were not *andriana*, the *mpanjaka* of the Zafindraraoto lineage was not regarded as a *mpitan-tranobe*, but was recognized as guarding the sacred wood of his lineage.

During my fieldwork, the position of *mpitan-tranobe* was held by Liva. Liva was said to be in his 60s, a fact that led to much scandal when he, a widower, married a young woman of 16. When his house was destroyed in a cyclone in 1994, rather than having it rebuilt, he moved to a remote location some two kilometers distant, where he and his new bride established their own family in a lone hilltop house surrounded by sugarcane and overlooking the mountains, a river, and the radiant green rice fields of his family.

"I left [the village] because there are so many *andevo* [slaves] in Ranotsara that no one is fit to guard the *hazomanga* [of the Zafinaraina lineage]," Liva explained.

The label of *andevo* is a strong one in Madagascar. To be descended from slaves marks one a social outcast, unsuitable for marriage among those of *hova* or *andriana* ancestry. While it is true that there came to be two classes of slaves in Madagascar, *andevo mainty* ["black" slaves, prohibited from marrying outside their caste, or owning land], and *andevo fotsy* ["white" slaves, similar to indentured servants who could buy their way out of servitude], any rumor of being descended from slaves is ruinous.

Yet Liva's allegation, while he would not elaborate, became an allegation I was to eventually hear repeatedly. Indeed, as more and more people of both lineages died, it became common rumor that the reason for the deaths was that there were so many *andevo* in the village. How is it, then, that Ranotsara, said to be founded by two lineages, one of free people who, as masters of the land, granted to the Zafinaraina prized agricultural lands, is now cast as a village of untouchables—a lineage descended from slaves—whose intermarriage with the royal Zafinaraina has cursed the village with sickness and death, and whose cohabitation with the royal descendants has rendered the original masters of the land landless—laboring for wages of approximately thirty cents a day on lands that they themselves are said to control?

This puzzle is at the heart of sickness and environmental change in Ranotsara.

Caste and Class in Ranotsara

As stated in the foregoing, the village was founded by two men—Rabiby, of the Zafinaraina lineage, and Ramanjato, of the Zafindraraoto lineage. Sometime around 1915 Rabiby's grandson, Ramitsiry, married Ramanjato's daughter, iKalahafa. Their youngest son, Tody, is one of the oldest men in the village, next in line to be *mpanjaka-be*, should his cousin Liva die before him. As such, Tody is respected as a *mpanjaka* in the village, while Liva lives *an-tsaha* (away, near his *tavy* fields).

The marriage of Tody's father, a Zafinaraina, to a woman of the Zafindraraoto lineage is said to have brought a curse to Ranotsara. Indeed, one well-respected elder alleges that the marriage was one of royalty to a slave—that iKalahafa was *andevo*, and by allowing such a marriage, and worse, burying Ramitsiry in his family's tomb despite his fall from grace, the village has been cursed ever since.

Things were hardly made better when two of Rabiby's grandaughters followed suit, with Nirina marrying Ramanjato's grandson Faly, and her sister Bely marrying Faly's brother Sabo.

Nirina is now an old woman; sometimes she says that she is seventy years old, other times she thinks that she is maybe ninety. She has a face woven in deep lines and a strong, straight body that moves slowly, as if in pain. Her eyesight is poor, she can no longer see the stones in the rice or the rats in the dark, but her eyes are alive. Her expressions change like lightning with more toothless grins and howling heckles than a cartoon character, her brain even more animated, and her arms and her back and her neck nearly as strong as any man's.

Nirina explains that she had known Faly since they were children, and they were always very close, although they grew up in separate villages. Because it was her mother who was Rabiby's daughter, Nirina was raised in her father's village, while she retained family ties to Ranotsara. When she grew up, she married a man she no longer speaks of, and they moved to several cities in Madagascar, including Tulear, a French colonial port. As such, Nirina became a woman of the world, and when her marriage ended in divorce, she returned to Ranotsara and married her childhood friend, Faly.

"My grandfather was one of the first men to build a home in Ranotsara when it was over there," she gestures toward the hills of the enclosed Ranomafana National Park. "Because of this, my family wanted me to guard the *hazo-manga*," she explained, referring to the succession of *mpanjaka*, "but I did not want the responsibility. So to appease the people, I married someone who could guard the *hazo-manga* for his own lineage. That is why I married Faly." Nirina's explanation for her marriage to Faly as merely for the sake of propriety was never very credible—they were extremely close, the best of drinking buddies who constantly joked and bickered among themselves with unashamed pride in each other. However, while it is not common, women can be chosen for the honor of *mpanjaka*, and so her comment is at least an interesting one.

Nirina and Faly had one child, who died in infancy. Nirina was unable to bear children afterwards, and so they adopted a son, Etienne, as their own.

"They never had any more children," an elder explained, "because the marriage was *fady* [taboo]. Nirina is *andriana-be* [very royal], her grandfather founded the village. She displeased the ancestors when she married an *andevo*."

Her sister Bely was said to have been equally cursed, not only losing an eye, which Bely said grew bigger and bigger until it exploded, but suffering from *salamanga* as well. *Salamanga* is a very rare spirit possession disorder, which, it is said in the neighboring village of Ambodiaviavy, afflicted her when she defied the ancestors yet again by failing to become an *ombiasa* as they wished for her. Her life in poverty and the many deaths of her family members were the prices she paid for transgressing the social order and marrying the descendent of a slave.

But did Nirina and Bely marry the descendents of slaves, as is commonly whispered in the village? Did Ramintsiry marry into the *andevo* cast as well? And does it really matter? I suggest that they did not marry into slavery—if, indeed, iKalahafa, Faly, and Sabo had been descended from slaves, the marriages would not have been allowed to take place, and when deceased, Raminstiry and Bely would not have been buried in their ancestral tomb afterwards, as they were (and the elders of the village concurred that Nirina will be buried among the Zafinaraina as well). And if the Zafindraraoto lineage was indeed descended from slaves, it is unlikely that they would have amassed so much land. Finally, and most importantly, there is no record of the Zafindraraoto lineage being anything but *hova*.[1]

Recasting the Zafindraraoto as *andevo*, however, might help to justify present economic relations in the village. Ramitsiry and iKalahafa had two sons and four daughters. The youngest son, Tody, is already one of the eldest men in the village, as has previously been mentioned. But their eldest son, Lahy, since passed away, married Sely, an elderly woman who wants as little to do with foreigners as possible, recalling very clearly the many waves of *vazaha* who have come to their village to "help," first during the colonial years when she was a young mother in Ranotsara, later with the Ministry of Forests and Water to control *tavy* farming, and most recently, with the Park. Now she lives with her youngest son and oversees the family's affairs, leaving it to them to deal with the outsiders.

For reasons that remain unclear, Lahy had been selected by the colonial officers in the region to receive coffee and banana trees. As such, he not only had the cash-crop colonial concessions to control, he had also been in a position to purchase many cattle, and to hire highland migrants to work his fields. These factors alone do not account for the current status of his family, but did lay a foundation.

Lahy and Sely had three sons and three daughters. As the eldest, Koto received the best farming lands of his family. Among these lands were many irrigated rice fields, passed on from his ancestors, who, as Zafinaraina, had received the flat lands from the *tompon-tany* [masters of the land], the Zafindraraoto. Koto managed these lands with care, and re-

---

1. Hanson (personal communication 1999) who has conducted extensive historical research of the area, including the Zafindraraoto lineage, has also indicated to me that he has never heard of this lineage being associated with *andevo*.

ceived many cattle from his father which he also managed with care. He also cleared his own *tavy* fields, and as his cash resources increased, he purchased land from others in Ranotsara. As discussed in the previous chapter, the sale of land was not customary; nonetheless, as the shift to cash crops contributed to a decline in subsistence crops and economic differentials, it became more common for land to be sold during cash shortages.

Koto's youngest brother, Rivo, was similarly positioned with favorable lands and many cattle. The brothers were both blessed with keen business sense, the willingness and energy to work hard, and the particularly useful skill of working well with outsiders.

Their sister, Baovita, had a son, Pascal, who the brothers soon recognized shared their entrepreneurial vision and even spoke a bit of French. While he did not have the lands or cattle of the two brothers, Pascal's outgoing personality, business sense, and best of all, his marriage to Rahasoa, a school teacher, provided him with the essential access to outside channels that the brothers needed to take advantage of outside resources and the ever in-coming *vazaha*.

Another brother, Lita, received prize lands from his father, and worked as hard as his brothers. But as his eyesight began to fade and blindness sealed his fate, Lita kept more and more to himself. Unable to engage in business, unable to work, it was left to his wife, Soa, and their eldest children, Ketaka, Chantelle and Lala, to farm the lands.

Eventually, Soa and the children could not maintain the irrigated rice production. In the generations past, these responsibilities would be shared by other family members. But in the recent years, the rapid inflation, accompanied by a number of cyclones, led to rice and cash shortages. These factors, integrally linked to structural adjustment policies and an in-flux of international development projects, enabled the three men to capitalize on the economic changes affecting the village.

Koto describes these years, from 1985 to 1987, and again in the early 1990s, as a difficult period when his own economic situation declined, and he became further frustrated when he broke his back and could no longer work his fields. As such, he was forced to sell all of his cattle, and he transferred his lands to his children. His son, Philippe, a young but equally sharp business man, took his place managing the family lands.

Koto indicated that it was during these years that people throughout the village stopped helping each other out. "In the past, if someone died, everyone contributed to the cost of the cow or rice. Now, only the family contributes. This changed during my generation; from my father's generation, only Tody is still living."

In the mid to late 1980s, as rising prices (associated with structural adjustment, the Gulf War, and the influx of *vazaha* with the coming of the park) and severe cyclones led to rice and cash shortages, Rivo, Pascal, and Philippe helped the villagers by loaning rice and cash, in exchange for repayment in double the following year. As such, many people found themselves in debt to the three men, while the three men grew prosperous.

When the *vazaha* came to Ranomafana to construct the JIRAMA dam, the three men, led by Rivo, organized village men to construct housing for the outsiders. And when the park project came to the village, as will be discussed subsequently, the two brothers were among the first to accept the new policies, rallying to receive the outsiders. Their seeming eagerness to embrace the new policies and embark on new farming techniques, along with Ranotsara's close proximity to the forest and its relative proximity to Ranomafana, made the village appear particularly appealing to the project officials and so it was subsequently selected as a pilot village of the project. By being designated a pilot village, the residents were assured that through assistance to these open-minded men, they would receive development assistance in the form of fish for stocking fish ponds, beans for a woman's cooperative, cement and roofing for the school, and seeds for farming irrigated rice. With Rivo, Philippe, Pascal and his wife, Rahasoa, taking charge of distribution, these resources, often intended for the benefit of all the residents, remained a subject of village gossip as to where the products ended up.

As people could no longer keep up with the spiraling cost of living, and as their rice was being used to repay prior years' debts, they were no longer able to produce enough rice and other crops to survive. Consequently, according to a number of villagers who rented out their lands, Rivo, Pascal, and Philippe, offered landholders up to 50,000FMG (approximately $12.50 at the time of my fieldwork) to rent their fields for a period of three years.[2]

This plan was most logical for those of the Zafindraraoto lineage because not being related to the four men of the Zafinaraina lineage, they could receive, along with the cash advance, the opportunity to continue working the fields for daily wages of up to 30 cents a day, plus a daily meal. This strategy enabled the most impoverished residents to ensure their survival, while not entirely relinquishing their rights to their land, which they could receive three years later when times were better or, if no better, renew the lease for additional cash. It further enabled Rivo, Pascal, Koto, and Philippe, to manage the dirty business of securing fertilizers, chemical inputs, seeds, and other goods from the *vazaha*. By working for the four men, the villagers were assured that rather than being

---

2. One informant indicated to me that if a person failed to repay the debt, the lender would take the person's land. This comment was not corroborated, nor was it clear if the land would be permanently or temporarily seized. I neither doubt the statement nor disregard it, without further evidence.

subjected to the rule of outsiders, the outsiders would provide resources to the village, because Rivo, Pascal, and Philippe knew exactly how to negotiate with this old breed. And, no matter the unequal access to resources these men had, they remained family (intermarriage having cast everyone in some type of obligatory relationship); there are limits to the domination family members can exercise over each other, whereas history had shown that no such limits extended to *vazaha*.

Thus, while so many of the Zafindraraoto lineage surrendered their lands, if only temporarily, those of the Zafinaraina lineage did not necessarily need to do the same, because by sending one or two sons or daughters to help out on their relative's land, they were supporting their relatives' growing wealth, and in so doing, indirectly ensuring their own future protection. After all, in a village of thirty households, there weren't many fields held by the Zafinaraina lineage that didn't already belong to one of these four men or their immediate family.

But not all of the Zafinaraina lineage could afford the luxury of retaining their land. Some, such as Lita's family, simultaneously rented out their lands, and provided gratuitous child labor so that they could benefit from both the immediate cash provisions of renting out land, and the long-term protective welfare promised by the kin network.

As the Zafindraraoto rented out more and more of their fields, or worked as wage laborers for the Zafinaraina men, it came to be that in every Zafindraraoto household there were no longer enough people to work the fields that were not rented. It is in this way that the majority of the land and labor shifted from the Zafindraraoto to the Zafinaraina and, I believe, that the recasting of the Zafindraraoto from *hova* to *andevo* began to be whispered about the village.

Another significant change linked to the international economy contributed to land consolidation in Ranotsara. From 1993 to 1994, the national government promoted land titling in the Ranomafana region (Hanson 1997) — in accordance with World Bank efforts to privatize land holdings and thereby presumably encourage conservation (see Keck, Sharma and Feder 1994; Leisz, Robles and Gage 1994). Hanson (1997) suggests that the land in the Ranomafana region that was registered with Madagascar's *Service de Domain* under this privatizing campaign was almost all wet rice fields.

That fewer *tavy* fields were registered might be explained by the registration requirements. In order to title land, the petitioner must have the land surveyed and mapped (Keck, Sharma and Feder 1994), a difficult process in a community where access to land surveyors and the money to pay them is short. In addition, it is not sufficient that one request title to property; it must also be shown that the land has been actively used for agricultural production for ten years, though in some cases this may be reduced to five years (Keck, Sharma and Feder 1994:15). Hence, gaining title to one's *tavy* fields may prove problematic if the land has been left fallow. Finally, because in order to register land, one must pay an initial registration fee and annual taxes, only those with the most cash income are likely to participate.

Rivo, Philippe, and Pascal, the three men whose control of community resources had expanded with the economic and social changes of the 1980's, were in the forefront of privatizing land during the early 1990's. Rahefa recalls how the land he had inherited from his father, Faralahy, was lost in this way. Before Faly became the *mpanjaka* of the Zafindraraoto lineage in Ranotsara, his elder brother, Faralahy held the position. Faralahy passed on some of his *tanim-bary* [irrigated rice land] to one of his sons, Rahefa; the remainder of his land he sold to Philippe when the economic crisis of the late 1980s impoverished him. Rahefa went *an-tsaha*, that is, he went to farm some distant *tavy* fields, and while gone, he rented his irrigated rice field to Rivo. Rahefa alleges that Rivo then registered the land in his own name; when Rahefa returned to Ranotsara, he said that he discovered he no longer owned the *tanim-bary*. Rahefa indicated that although there are indigenous methods of arbitration through the *fokonolona*, he decided not to challenge Rivo, due to the latter's wealth. He indicated that he feared Rivo's position in the village and that the Zafinaraina lineage had become much more powerful than Rahefa's own family of Zafindraraoto *mpanjaka*.

Others in the village echoed this concern. For example, Liva, *mpanjaka-be* of the Zafinaraina lineage, reported that the strength of the *mpanjaka* was diminishing, and that this decline began during his brother's reign as *mpanjaka* (I am not sure when his brother assumed the position of *mpanjaka*, but he died sometime around 1993). As an example of how power was shifting in the community, Liva indicated that when I arrived in the village and asked permission to reside there, I was brought first to the home of Rivo, and later to the home of Pascal; it was these men who granted me permission to reside in the village. Rivo assumed authority in the matter of my residence, and acted as contractor for the building of my house. What he should have done, Liva indicated, was asked permission of him, as *mpanjaka-be*. He did not, because my residing in the village was viewed as an economic opportunity, and hence, the local entrepreneurs took charge.

Liva's report was certainly an accurate account of my experience. It was not until I had moved to the village and the house was completed that I was even told of Liva's position; while Faly and Tody were introduced to me as the *mpanjaka*, they took no initiative in any dialogue and deferred to Rivo, Faly later telling me that his own authority had significantly diminished with the emerging wealth and social skills (in dealing with *vazaha*) of Rivo.

Faly indicated that the role of the *mpanjaka* had changed in many ways in recent years. For example, he indicated that when he first became *mpanjaka*, if a person wanted to clear a new field, he could not do so until he first worked on the fields of the *mpanjaka*. Faly's son, Etienne, added that in past generations if a person wanted to clear a new field, they had to ask permission of the *mpanjaka*, but with the increasing land shortages of the last decade, they no longer asked permission, unless as a formality. "Now the land belongs to all the people," he said, suggesting that ancestral land associated with a lineage was disappearing in favor of a new type of common property regime which a select few have been controlling.

Rather than challenging the local appropriation of land and power, Faly and many others chose instead to accept it, in order to reap direct and indirect benefits in this period of social change. Faly told me that he felt he had very little power to change the situation, yet he recognized that Rivo and the others could provide a relatively reliable conduit to the resources of outsiders. By resisting the temptation to invoke his authority as *mpanjaka* and accuse Rivo and his kin of enriching themselves by appropriating resources (such as rice provided by the national government after the cyclone, beans provided by the project for a woman's cooperative, and materials provided by the project for repairing the local school), Faly and his wife, Nirina, chose to work with and for Rivo. By conferring unspoken approval upon the activities of the village's entrepreneurs, Faly was able to exercise continued and unchallenged authority over Rivo in non-economic matters of the village, avail himself of wage-work when needed, and not have to worry about dealing with *vazaha*.

In contrast, Rivo's own elder, Liva, left the village rather than continue in a role he found to be ceremonial only.[3] Tensions between himself and his kin continued, while he continued to invoke his authority as *mpanjaka-be* and elder of the Zafinaraina lineage in order to position himself close to those in real power, and more importantly for Liva, contrast his own lineage to that of Faly. Insisting that the Zafindraraoto were *andevo*, he maintained that his own position was the highest in the village and his own ancestry the most pure. Not only did he claim an historical right to his title as *mpanjaka-be*, by excluding himself from the village, distinguishing his lineage from that of Faly, and associating at a distance with Rivo whom he pointed out was descended from a union with *andevo*, Liva claimed a moral right to his title because he was one of the few in the village who remained uncontaminated by the lineage of the inferior "other."

---

3. Since leaving the village I have learned that Liva planned to return to the village because the ancestors had been displeased by his departure; he had hoped that in so doing, there might be fewer deaths.

Accessing Health Resources

In addition to seizing land and power in the village, the leading men of the Zafinaraina lineage have also assumed authority over health care in certain respects. While Rivo and Koto are respected for controlling an indigenous treatment for measles that is provided annually to the children of the village, Rivo and Pascal, by way of their frequent trips to Ranomafana, access to cash, facility with outsiders, and, for Pascal, marriage to the school teacher, have acted as spokesmen for the village in negotiating access to health services provided by the Ranomafana National Park Project. In this way the men of the community, rather than the women, have central roles in accessing Western health care, with the exception of Rahasoa, a school teacher whose position (and marriage to Pascal) have enabled her to play a strategic role in accessing, controlling, and dispensing medicines.

Men's physical strength is another factor contributing to their important role regarding health care. Because it is difficult to carry a sick child or adult across rivers and hills to reach health services in Ranomafana, Ifanadiana, or more distantly if necessary, men's work determines in many cases whether or not a person receives such care. For example, on many occasions Rivo or Pascal's frequent trips to Ranomafana included picking up medicines for themselves or others, or even carrying a sick or wounded person to the clinic. Conversely, to those who worked for wages, such a trip meant loss of income. There were a few occasions when I compensated a family for these lost wages so that a child or adult would get treatment promptly. Had I not done so, I am certain that the family would have delayed or disregarded treatment to avoid losing income that was so necessary to survival.

Despite the ability of certain men to access biomedical health services in Ranomafana and elsewhere—services which are appallingly inadequate and likely in many cases to worsen one's health—the poverty of everyone (for even the land rich residents have limited food and cash), combined with an unhealthy environment, extremely demanding work loads and geographical isolation, contribute to poor health for all village residents. Yet, the consolidation of economic power has enabled certain village residents to maintain a ready supply of pharmaceutical medicines for treating respiratory disorders and fevers, while the rapid decline in economic status of most residents, and the associated decline in their nutritional and health status, has contributed to a growing dependency upon forest and local indigenous medicines for others in treating these same illnesses, though they are more likely to seek treatment only when these illnesses become acute or interfere with work. Chronic illnesses, however, are more likely to be minimally treated, if at all. Moreover, differences in age, gender, and religion have also shaped how health resources are viewed and obtained.[4]

To understand how health and healing are conceptualized differently by residents within the same village, and how lineage has become fundamental to these differences, I turn again to history with a discussion of how twentieth century land and social changes, discussed in Chapters Four and Five, have shaped health and health care in the forest regions of Madagascar.

Changes in Health and Health Care

The population of Madagascar had declined significantly throughout the late nineteenth century, and this decline was tied first to the *fanompoana* labor of the Merina autocracy (leading to famine and disease) (Campbell 1992), and second, to the colonial insurrection (Antananarivo Annual 1898). Campbell (1992) indicates that the declining population of the late nineteenth century was preceded by a fifty per cent annual fatality rate among soldiers of the imperial (Merina) army, and several smallpox epidemics from the early and mid-1830s. These losses were primarily centered in the highlands, but contributed to population migrations to forested and coastal regions as people sought to escape servitude, death and illness. The losses of the latter part of the century, however, were more far-reaching, affecting people in the lower highlands, particularly those now identified as "Betsileo", as well as the forested regions where rice production declined. Campbell (1992) notes that the pre-colonial autocracy of the Merina empire contributed to the population losses associated with colonialism. Challenging the view that the violence and social dislocation associated with foreign incursions into Africa created such ecological disturbance that catastrophic human and animal diseases ensued, Campbell argues that natural causes only partly account for disease and famine in Madagascar during the late nineteenth century. More salient, he suggests, is the extreme *fanompoana* labor imposed during the precolonial Merina autocracy. This cycle of disease and famine also contributed to demographic change.

.... The birth rate in Madagascar.... was profoundly upset by the adoption of *fanompoana* from the mid-1820s. *Fanompoana* decreased income opportunities for young adults, which probably resulted in a rise in the average age of marriage and

---

4. These points are examined more thoroughly in Chapters Seven and Eight.

in depressed fertility, and it involved long periods of harsh physical labour, with inadequate rations, which delayed puberty and altered ovulatory cycles in women, thus depressing fertility, as well as increasing the incidence of miscarriages (Nurse, Weiner & Jenkins 1985:253-254). Traditionally, women worked harder than men and their burden increased from the adoption of autarky, notably in the gold fields from the 1880s (Campbell 1988a, 1988b, 1988c). Thirdly, the frequency of conception was reduced as *fanompoana* often separated men and women and, in order to spare the future generation from *fanompoana* some couples probably limited their family size through practising abortion and, despite the royal ban, infanticide. Decary (1947-48:30) and Sibree (1924:253) estimate that infanticide was responsible for the deaths of 14.29 and 25 per cent respectively of Malagasy babies (Campbell 1992:420, 421).

Campbell further suggests that the spread of *fanompoana* labor contributed to the rapid spread of venereal diseases, particularly in male labor camps, and to women's increasing employment in prostitutition.

As in mainland Africa, the declining health of the Malagasy people was of great concern to the colonial state. Because colonial labor policies necessitated an abundant and healthy labor pool, demographic factors such as population losses, either from death or migration, were directly linked to political concerns.

Therefore, to augment the shrinking population in order that the labor pool available to the colonial state be steady throughout the twentieth century, the colonial government established medical hospitals, dispensaries for Western pharmaceuticals, and medical schools for training Malagasy (urban, elite Merina) in biological theories and treatments of disease, including an emphasis on improved hygiene to improve health and reproductive fitness. The Antananananarivo Annual, a nineteenth century journal published by the London Missionary Society, described in detail the colonial objectives of increasing the Malagasy population. Central to this policy was a form of social engineering, in which the Merina (aka Hova) of the highlands were identified as a distinct race which was superior to the populations of the coastal regions.

> The first matter noticed is the small amount of the population of Madagascar compared with the great extent of the island, there being probably only 6.6 inhabitants to a square kilometre. The next point is, that the Hova race appears to be the only one capable of furnishing the population of the future and sufficient manual labour. "In one word, it is the Hova race which is the superior one of Madagascar, the one which, by its com-

mercial instincts, its desire for comfort and its love of gain, and its ability to work, is destined to spread itself more and more over the entire island, to absorb the other peoples, and to give our colonists intelligent and trained assistants, if we take all the necessary measures to encourage the development of this population."...In order to promote the fecundity of the Hova race, which seems an undoubted fact in the past, the General proposes to use a number of different measures; and these he groups under five heads, as follows:—(1) legal, (2) administrative, (3) hygienic, (4) political, and (5) fiscal (Antananarivo Annual 1898:247, quote uncited).

Legal measures included promotion of exogamy and inter-caste marriages, fines for divorce, and "the strict application of punishment" (ibid:247) against women practicing abortion. Moreover, as *fanompoana* gave way to "prestation" or unremunerated labor for the colonial government, all men "legally" married were exempt from service if they had five or more children, while "young Hovas legally married and the fathers of one child will be exempted from military service" (Antananarivo Annual 1898:248), and families with at least seven children were provided with free education for one of these children. Men who reached the age of 25 years and women of 21, and who were not married, were taxed. Moreover, a "Children's Fete" was instituted in which large families were honored, with money and gifts presented to such families and the parents provided with "prominent positions" (Antananarivo Annual 1898:248). In these ways, the colonial government promoted early marriage and large families.

Another important administrative measure taken to increase the agricultural labor supply was to promote *tavy* production. Attributing the abolition of slavery to declining agricultural labor as freed-slaves became porters, the colonial state took the position that tying people to land would promote agricultural production:

> Owing to the rapid formation of roads practicable for carriages, porters' work will gradually be less needed; and it will be desirable to increase the number of natives who hold land. In all cases, however, holders must be obliged to cultivate (Antananarivo Annual 1898:248).

Finally, increasing the health of the Malagasy was considered paramount to augmenting the labor supply.

> Under the heading of *hygienic and medical measures*, it is noticed that notwithstanding the efforts of the various missions, the laws of health are still very imperfectly understood by the

Malagasy, especially as shown by their non-use of warm clothing in the cold season of the year, the want of sanitary arrange-
ments, and the prevalence of certain diseases. The causes of
sterility, and of the high rate of infant mortality, are pointed
out, as well as remedies for this in the spreading of medical
knowledge, and the formation of hospitals, dispensaries, and
medical schools. Drunkenness should be severely punished; and
it is necessary that popular and simple tracts on medicine and
hygiene should be prepared and widely circulated among the
people.

Campbell (1992) indicates that the introduction of Western medicine
through the Protestant missionary societies (who used the new medicine
as a bargaining chip to convert people to Christianity) and its promotion
by the colonial government, had significant effects on the use of indigenous medicine as well. In the mid-nineteenth century, as *fanompoana* labor
led to widespread death and disease, and as traditional medicine proved
inadequate to combat such health problems, many Malagasy were drawn
to the health care services being introduced by the missionaries.

But after 1870, several social and natural events contributed to an even
sharper increase in death and disease. The population circulations associated with *fanompoana* labor, in which people from the malarial zones of
the coasts and forests moved freely in and out of the highlands, brought
malaria epidemics to the highlands. In addition, as men were forced to
labor for others, their own irrigated rice fields were often left idle, creating breeding grounds for the anopheles mosquito in the lowlands. Finally,
unusually wet weather made an additional contribution to rising malaria
epidemics throughout the island. Another factor which Campbell points
to as facilitating the spread of disease during this period was the introduction of new disease brought by European steamships as trade between
the Merina kingdom and Europe increased.

Among the people of the southern highlands, impoverishment and
famine were compounded by particularly cold winters for which the people lacked adequate clothing, leading to severe respiratory infections. As the
"Betsileo" region was particularly hard hit, many groups migrated toward
the southeastern forested regions.

Campbell (1992:422-424) comments on the effects of this migration:

> This combination of climatic and dietary factors, accentu-
> ated in forced labour camps by insanitary conditions, facilitated
> the spread of disease.... Thus, in overall terms, a plateau envi-
> ronment traditionally considered healthy was, from the late
> 1870s, transformed into one wracked by unrelenting disease
> and famine. This change, following hard upon the adoption of

Christianity as the imperial religion, tested to the limit the ability of the latter, in the form of its preventative and curative prescriptions, to meet the crisis. Of notable importance in this were Western medicines and the *taratasy* [paper, in this instance, the Bible], the most powerful of Christian talismans.

Because the new medicine could not combat the escalating death and disease, many Malagasy returned to using indigenous medicines, but rather than abandoning one form of medicine for the other, they integrated the new European medicines and biomedical ideas with the indigenous pharmacopeia to increase the medical options available to them (Campbell 1992:35). Rather than perceiving the curative power to be inherent in the medicine, however, successful cures were attributed to the power of the indigenous healer. This resurgence of faith in indigenous healing coincided with a revival in "traditional" ceremonial rites related to health and well being, as well as an increase in spirit possession.

D. Peters (1994a), however, points out that while missionaries condemned the practice of indigenous medicine, particularly the role of the *ombiasa* in health care, the Protestant and Catholic churches differed in their responses to those who continued to practice indigenous health care. Speaking specifically about the Ranomafana region, Peters notes that the Catholic church is the oldest church in the area, whereas the Lutheran church has been gaining greater popularity in recent years. With its own reverence for icons and chanting during worship, the Catholic church did not overtly condemn the practice of *ombiasa*. As such, Catholicism provided a greater opportunity for syncretic medicine to be practiced.

Conversely, the Lutheran church openly condemned the practice of *ombiasa* and forbade its followers from seeking treatment from indigenous healers, while promoting religious-based healing sessions as an alternative to *ombiasa*. D. Peters (1994a) notes that rather than being successful in this effort, people began visiting indigenous healers covertly, and insisting to outsiders that they did not practice indigenous medicine.

As these shifting strategies toward maintaining health care paralleled the demographic distribution of disease, the political and administrative policies of the colonial government to augment the labor pool proved effective. By 1941, however, the increasing population contributed to a shortage of rice. This was because reproductive control of men and women, accompanied by the introduction of Western drugs, vaccines, and health clinics, brought larger families and lower mortality. At the same time, the focus on cash crop production left less land available for subsistence rice production. To offset the impoverishment associated with the rice shortages and subsequent revolt in 1947, *tavy* production was intensified (Hanson 1997).

Free Western medicines, well-supplied health clinics, and Western-trained health practitioners remained available to the Malagasy of the Ranotsara/Ranomafana region throughout the colonial years. With liberation from colonial control, however, these services were reduced. By the late 1970s, they were further reduced when the Democratic Socialist Republic of Didier Ratsiraka shifted its social policies to the urban sector, at the neglect of the rural sector. Structural adjustment policies of the mid-1980s further limited funding available to the rural health sector. As such, by the late 1980s when the Ranomafana National Park Project made its appearance in Ranotsara, via a visit from the Principal Investigator for the project, the residents were eager to accept the health services she assured would come their way.

Older residents, who had been born and raised during the period of colonial rule, were among the most resistant to further encroachment on their land and lives by outsiders, but also the most enthusiastic about receiving the type of health care they had once been accustomed. Granted, the relative isolation of their village, their low social and economic status, and their alienation from colonial agents, influenced the quality of the health care they had received during those years, but unlike their younger relations, they had become familiar with the rapid and effective cure many Western medicines had provided them. Women, who had been the targets of maternal health services[5] were also among the most anxious for "modern" health services for their granddaughters. Both men and women, however, shared a strong desire for strong and efficacious medicines for their babies and children. Younger people, who had been born and raised during the 1970s and 1980s, had far less experience with such medicines, however. For them and their babies, sickness was a way of life.

The age and gender distinctions influencing one's view of medicines, and more importantly, the history of land appropriation, forced labor, cash-crop production, migration and reproductive control, played no part in the health research initiated by the Project. Indeed, as one anthropologist involved in the Project's first health survey indicated to me, her repeated appeals to project administrators to disregard ethnicity in favor of exploring more salient historical and social correlates to health, were completely dismissed and her own efforts to do so cut short with her termination from the project (Hardenbergh 1998, personal communication).

5. According to two older women, very few of the older women had ever given birth at home, recalling (with ambivalence) hospitalized births they found much safer, if not consistent with their indigenous beliefs. In contrast, only one woman of child-bearing age acknowledged to me that she had had a hospital birth, all others giving birth on the dirt floors of their homes.

Conceptualizing Ethnicity and Health

Prior to and during its first phase of the project (1990 to 1993), the project sought to gain cultural understandings relative to health care through the collection of sociocultural baseline data. Hanson (1997) argues that it was in the methodology of this data collection effort that categories of ethnicity became set in stone. He suggests that attempts to accumulate data on "households" were based on assumptions of what constituted "typical" "Betsileo" and "Tanala" households.

> In almost every one of these studies, resident peoples were first constructed along ethnic lines. Thus, people were defined as being of either the Betsileo or Tanala ethnic group... Building upon this ethnic basis, a set of standard sociological categories were used to further define the household, its occupants, and their role in local and more global markets.... (Hanson 1997:90).

In conjunction with this data collection effort, and not at all clearly separate in the views of most villagers, the project promised health care to the residents of the original 26 pilot villages surrounding the park. This health care was represented as a traveling health team, consisting of a physician, nurses, and midwives, who would diagnose and treat illnesses and injuries, and provide pharmaceutical medicines. To the residents, the link between the park and their health was that if they gave up their land, they would receive much-needed health services as compensation. To the project, however, it was necessary to establish a link between the objective of conservation and the strategy of development. By the time the second phase of the project was being designed, the link was achieved through a focus on control of reproduction. The Director of Conservation during the project's second phase was adamant on this point in his personal communications to me (1995-1996; recorded in field notes), suggesting that the only responsibility of the project in the area of health care was to control population growth so that *tavy* would decline.

As "Tanala" farmers were considered the primary *tavy* farmers, the objective of the project became to control reproduction of "Tanala" women. Under the guise of providing maternal and neo-natal health care, the project employed "midwives" who had no training in prenatal or neonatal care, or in delivering babies. They were trained to dispense birth control pills and condoms. Indeed, when a physician and midwife came to Ranotsara during my residency there, I requested the "midwife" to visit a woman who had given birth earlier in the week. The midwife responded, "Why?" I explained that the woman wasn't feeling well, and the baby should be examined. She declined the visit, she explained, because the woman, having just delivered, had no need for birth control.

Throughout the physician's visit, he received no assistance from the midwife, whose sole role was to wait for men and women to seek her out for birth control information. Four women did so, each receiving a one-month supply of birth control pills. They laughed, knowing full well that the "midwife" would not return with additional pills, and they were correct, despite my request to her that she do so.

In fact, when she visited the neighboring village of Moratoky, following her introduction to the community she began a lecture, in a scolding tone, to the villagers, telling them that the reason they were poor and the reason there were so many sick among them was because they had too many babies.

The selection of Ranotsara as a pilot village did bring with it health care for a few years. But internal divisions (associated with the rising economic power of the men of the Zafinaraina lineage) made the conservation and development objectives of the project difficult to carry out, and health care was abruptly stopped. While project administrators found local disagreements too problematic to continue agricultural assistance (and hence, health care—presented to the villagers as tied to relinquishing forest land and not to accepting agricultural assistance, was disregarded), the villagers perceived the abrupt and unexplained termination of health services as a "punishment" for their disobedient style of participation in the project—a participation which was at times at odds with how the project expected them to participate.

The internal divisions of the village forged its social identity as "Tanala", as rising economic and social inequalities led to intensified *tavy* production. Contrary to the belief that by encouraging the expansion of wet-rice fields, *tavy* production would decrease, it was found that *tavy* was not abandoned at all; it was merely augmented by increased wet-rice production (Ferraro 1994). In Ranotsara, it was those who had been provided with agricultural assistance by the project who most rapidly expanded their *tavy* fields, because they had been economically empowered to hire laborers and rent *tavy* fields from their less advantaged kin and neighbors.

The increasing impoverishment of the majority of residents served to reinforce an *image* of poverty, by way of visible markers such as inadequate and ragged clothing, dilapidated housing, and poor health and nutrition. This image of poverty was perceived by many outsiders as evidence of backwardness, ignorance, and laziness. The solidifying of a "Tanala" ethnic identity, which I believe was brought about in part by internal divisions in the village and in part by the project reifying 19th century stereotypes, contributed to the project abandoning the community as a pilot village. This abandonment was ironic given that being identified as "Tanala" was a primary factor in gaining access to health care because to be "Tanala" was presumed to mean being a *tavy* farmer and having too many children.

Hanson (1997:24,245) points to future conceptualizations of "Tanala" needs and the link between social identity and health:

> With the turn of the twenty-first century, the RNPP will in all likelihood be deeply involved in the lives of Ambodiaviavy residents. The question at this point is not whether RNPP planners will be able to introduce and define what they believe to be the true needs of the Tanala. This much is certain. Rather, the important consideration now is to what extent, the Tanala people of the Ranomafana region will be able to participate in this definition and interpretation process. This is no small matter. If we assume that a medical center, for example, is defined by the Project as a Tanala need, it will make a good deal of difference for the Tanala as to whether they decide who would staff the center, whether medical teams from the center reach Ambodiaviavy on a monthly basis, or whether the medicines within the center are offered to Tanala individuals free of charge or distributed to lineage leaders.

Hanson's concern for the "Tanala" residents of Ambodiaviavy is also a concern for the residents of Ranotsara. While Ranotsara is considered a "Tanala" village by the residents, most of whom describe themselves as descended from "Betsileo" ancestors, it has been identified in early project documents as a "Betsileo" village, which at the same time ranked the "Betsileo" heritage as superior to a "Tanala" ancestry. "To have both a Betsileo father and mother was a sign of distinction." [RNPP "Survey of Ranomafana Park Pilot Villages" 1989]. In contrast to the project's finding, not one of the residents I interviewed suggested that either ethnicity was superior to the other or that any distinction was conferred by having two "Betsileo" parents as opposed to one or none.

The village was also routinely described by project workers as a "Tanala" village during my residence there. The reason it was originally listed as a "Betsileo" village was that most of the residents, when asked their ethnic identity, are asked "*Inona no ny fokonao?*" which, roughly translated into English, is "What is your descent?" or "Who are your people?" As such, they indicate they are "Betsileo" because their ancestors were. Still, they persist in practicing *tavy*, thus conveying the "Tanala" status to project management. Moreover, as stated previously, the descent to greater and greater impoverishment has burned an image of backwardness and hopelessness into the eyes and hearts of project administration such that Ranotsara can now only be understood as "Tanala" to these outsiders.

Another important dimension to the way in which ethnicity is conceptualized, is reflected in the views of a local *ombiasa*, Naina. Naina is a handsome, well-built man in his late fifties, who has studied local medicines for at least thirty years, having learned most of them from his father, also an *ombiasa*. Naina, a widower who had lost most of his hearing, is now teaching the medicines to his son, Feno. Due to his hearing loss, he has become very dependent on Feno to be his ears for him. Unfortunately, while an eager student and very loyal to his father, sixteen-year-old Feno has already developed a heavy dependence on *toaka gasy*, and Naina is often at loss for assistance when Feno is unconscious from drink. Having no other son, and his older daughter showing more interest in boys than in medicines, Naina is concerned that Feno learn the medicines and not drink so much.

Naina explained that he was "Tanala," and the "Tanala," he suggested, unlike the "Betsileo," use medicines to treat illnesses of the head and stomach, and for general healing. The "Betsileo," although doing the same, he explained, are more likely to use medicines for ceremonies (as opposed to healing sickness), and also use medicines against their enemies. This distinction of "the other" as using medicines for ceremonies and sorcery was often made by *ombiasa*, regardless of their ethnic identification. They themselves claimed that they would never use medicines to harm, but others do, and others are defined in terms of ethnicity. The general consensus of the villagers, however, when talk turned to the subject of *ombiasa* and *mpamosavy* (witches), was that all *ombiasa* are learned in the arts of medicine, and know which plants heal and which harm, and they can all be hired to employ that knowledge to harm as well as hurt, whether they called themselves *mpamosavy* or not. Thus, while *ombiasa* are honored for their healing powers, they are also regarded as potentially injurious. Naina, however, insisted (as did all *ombiasa*) that he used his knowledge only to heal, and this often includes healing the illnesses caused by ("Betsileo") *mpamosavy* or by angry ancestors.

Naina's insistence that he practices "Tanala" medicine was also revealing in that Naina indicated he, like Nirina, was "Betsileo" "a long time ago" [*taloha be*], and that he had learned his craft from his "Betsileo" father. Nonetheless, having lived in Ranotsara all his life and practiced the "Tanala" way of living, which in Naina's case includes farming irrigated rice fields and *tavy*, as well as raising cattle, Naina became "Tanala," and consequently, his healing, too, became regarded as "Tanala." More significantly, in practice, it was not the "Betsileo" he regarded as his rivals; local competition among healers within the region surrounding Ranotsara led *ombiasa* to safeguard their healing secrets from their neighbors. In Naina's case, this positioned him in competition with both Rakoto, an *ombiasa* in Ranotsara, and Alarobia, an *ombiasa* and *mpanjaka* in nearby Moratoky. Both men are members of the same lineage as Naina, the Zafinaraina lineage, and all three descend from "Betsileo" ancestors.

The question then remains, if, to the residents, "Tanala" is a way of life, and "Betsileo" an ancestry, what exactly is the "Tanala" way of living? To the project, it is the practice of *tavy*; agricultural strategy is the boundary, and tied to the way that one farms the land is a host of other social values, including cleanliness, intellect, modernization, sexuality, superstition, and willingness to work.

To the residents, the "Tanala" way of living is the practice of *tavy*, as well as cash-crop production, irrigated rice farming, burial in caves, eating a diet of rice, greens, beans, manioc, and green bananas, giving birth at home, brewing and drinking *toaka gasy*, and recognizing and giving homage to the ancestors of the forest region. *Tavy*, to the residents of this "Tanala" village, is but one dimension of a complex economic and social system in which people attempt to support themselves and their families on a limited land-base constrained by the critical limitations of the forest environment; that is to say, heavy rains, cyclones, relatively infertile soils, steep terrain, and limited acces to markets and roads. The economy is dismal; W. J. Peters (1999, fn), citing Samisoa (1992), indicates that "In a random-sample survey of 100 village households in the Ranomafana National Park peripheral zone, 50 percent of all households (average size approximately 6 people/household) were found to have annual incomes from all sources of less than $50.00."

Contrary to the project image that to be "Tanala" was to be a *tavy* farmer and to be "Betsileo" was to be an irrigated farmer, in the village of Ranotsara, where the wealthier residents all owned both irrigated and tavy fields, and the poorer residents sold or rented their *tavy* and irrigated fields to the wealthier residents, there was no relationship between being "Betsileo" and practicing wet-rice agriculture, and being "Tanala" and practicing *tavy*. People practiced agriculture based upon the type of land and labor available to them, not based on "the way of the ancestors" or their ethnic identity.

Most importantly, there are not two different agricultural systems managed by two different types of people. There exists a single agricultural system which includes horticultural elements. That is to say, the people practice swidden and irrigated agriculture concurrently, along with cash-crop production.

A common view of the persistence of *tavy* is that it is a form of resistance (e.g. Bryant and Bailey 1997; Hanson 1997; Jarosz 1993).

> A comparable [to "scientific forestry" in Java] record of everyday resistance occurred in colonial Madagascar where, as Jarosz (1993) shows, French colonial officials sought to stamp out shifting cultivation, but in the process only incurred the implacable opposition of shifting cultivators in this colony. Shifting cultivation (or *tavy*) was a form of long-term land management used for centuries by the Malagasy, but concerns about

the possible adverse effects of such cultivation on the island's commercially valuable forests prompted the French to ban this practice in those forests in 1913. As elsewhere in the colonial world (Bryant, 1994a; Jewitt, 1995), this policy was linked to a paternalistic quest to 'civilise' shifting cultivators through a sedentarisation programme that aimed to convert hill-dwelling cultivators into valley-dwelling commercial farmers. However, this 'colonial vision proved difficult to implement' as a result of the widespread resistance of the Malagasy to the restrictions placed on the *tavy* (Jarosz, 1993:375). Everyday resistance here, as in Dutch-ruled Java, often involved nothing more than the perpetuation of practices that were now illegal, and shifting cultivators were arrested or forced to pay fines for burning and clearing state-protected forests. Indeed, the *tavy* represented a conscious quest to hold on to local culture and beliefs; the fact that such cultivation was undertaken in traditional dress and using traditional tools was a piquant rejection of French attempts to convert the Malagasy to a more 'civilised' European way of life (Jarosz, 1993) (Bryant and Bailey 1997:171, 172).

I would suggest that rather than conceptualizing *tavy* as a form of cultural resistance, which it may well be, it may be more useful to focus on how—and which—people do *not* resist intervention. While *tavy* may persist, many people do indeed embrace agricultural innovations (while not abandoning *tavy*) and economic change. Who is positioned to do so, and how they strategize such changes, illuminates the internal social differences that homogenized concepts of cultural belief systems fail to flesh out.

In the following chapter I shift from the discussion of *tavy* and history, to consider how the daily lives and environment of the residents of Ranotsara are experienced bodily. Encircled by wet-rice fields, in which they labor daily, backs bent and knee deep in fecal-contaminated water, cooking over open fires in small, windowless rooms, sharing bed and closet-sized homes with five or six family members, eating minimally and working exhaustively to provide the necessities of life, sickness is hard and lasting for many. This sickness, viewed as "natural" when cast as "tropical" illnesses, is shared by all, regardless of status. Gender and age, however, mediate the types of illnesses which strike, and cash resources influence treatment. Nonetheless, illness and disease in Ranotsara are associated with the social changes of migration, increased labor, housing, agricultural practices, and animal husbandry, suggesting that there is nothing natural about tropical sickness. What has become naturalized to the residents, however, is the suffering of the body, the chronic discomfort one internalizes from infancy, when scabies afflicts a newborn at two weeks of age, intestinal parasites infest the crawling baby, malaria sickens the toddler, and chronic coughing strikes the child. By adulthood, when breathing is difficult and walking is painful, one has learned sickness and ache as a "natural" condition. The following chapter will show how this naturalized sickness is experienced and accepted.

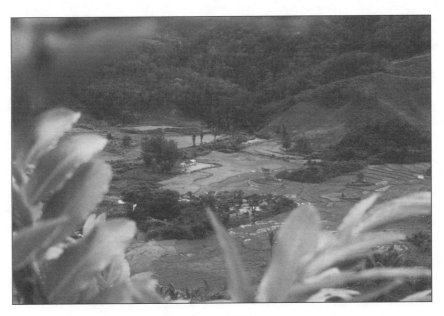

The village of Ranotsara.

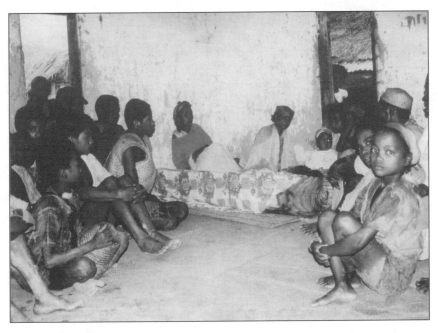

Villagers attend the corpse of a young woman who has died.

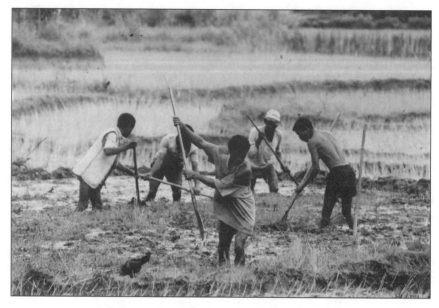

Men prepare a field for planting irrigated rice.

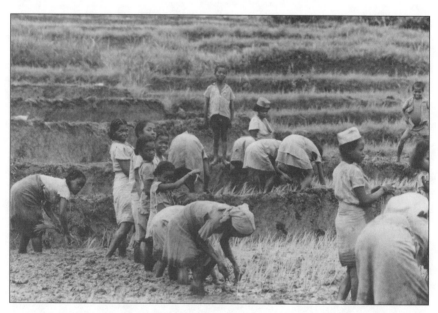

Young girls plant rice in an irrigated rice field.

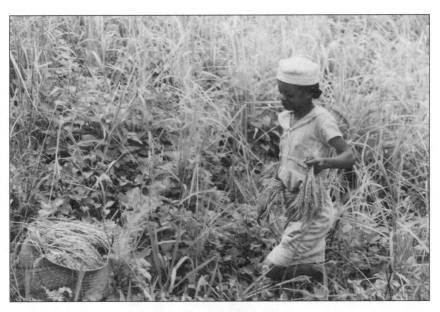

A woman bringing in her tavy harvest.

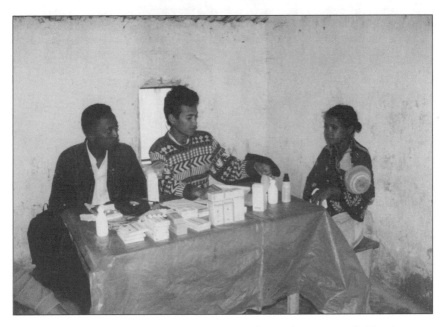

Soa brings her newborn baby to Dr. Tovo for medicines provided by the
Malagasy national airlines and a national pharmaceutical company.

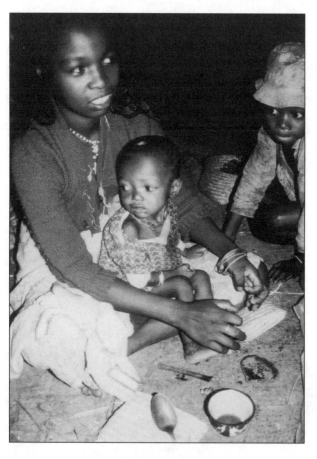

A woman applies a paste made from wild ginger root to her son's head and limbs to protect him from malevolent spirits.

Chapter 7

Naturalizing Sickness

Medicine for the Dead

My first day in the village was spent unpacking my far too many provisions, arranging someone to help with the cooking (a young woman named Lalao), and someone to help with the laundry (an older woman named Patrisse), as well as meeting many people. It was a busy, stressful day that ended with my feeling more like Lucy Ricardo than Margaret Mead. Finally, however, the introductions had been made, I had been warmly welcomed, and my desk and bed were in place. Several women joined me for my first meal, and the dishes were washed in the river. As the women were bidding me goodnight and I was longing for privacy once more, there was a knock at the door. I answered it, and in the darkness I discerned a young, timid woman, late in pregnancy, holding out a note for me.

The note was written by Jacqueline, a woman from Ranomafana who had assisted me with finding a village for my research. I translated the note from French to English as I read it to myself in the dim candlelight,

"Madame Janezi," Jacqueline wrote, "This is Nety. She is from Ranotsara. She can cook and clean and help you in many ways. She needs a job. Please hire her."

I did not know what to do. I did not need a cook, or anyone to clean my home.

"I would like to hire you," I attempted to say in my pathetic rendition of the "Tanala" dialect, "but I do not need anyone. I already have someone to cook, and someone to do laundry, and a research assistant."

She looked heartbroken. She probably needed an income very badly, and being pregnant and female, I wondered if she had any land or laborers to assist her with farming. As young as she was, in her late teens or early twenties, it was also quite possible she had no husband.

I looked around the room, and saw the piece of foam wrapped in sheets and blankets, which was my bed. I recalled another anthropologist telling me that he hired a woman to make his bed and sweep the floors, just because she needed the money.

"You could make my bed. I could pay you to make my bed and sweep the floors," I suggested, knowing it made me sound incredibly elitist to hire someone to do something I could so obviously do for myself.

"What would the salary be?" she asked, clearly unimpressed with the job.

I had been told by many people that I had been paying my research assistant, and any others I hired for whatever job, far too much for the local economy and it was creating conflicts. Consequently, I vowed that no matter how absurdly low the local wages, I would start paying within the limits of the local economy. So I quoted her a price, I don't recall how much, one that was low but relative to the wages I was paying for Lalao to cook and Patrisse to wash my clothes.

"That is not enough..." she said in a barely audible whisper as she looked to the floor. To admit that the pay was not enough was clearly difficult for her. A crowd of about fifteen or twenty people had surrounded us, and no matter my efforts to direct them out the door, this first night in Ranotsara was proving me to be ineffectual in a number of respects.

"I know that it is not enough to live on," I explained, "but it will only take five or ten minutes a day, and the pay will increase, and if I find more work, I can hire you for more." She continued to look devastated.

"*Tsy ampy izany, tsy ampy izany*" ["It is not enough"] she repeated, mostly to the floor.

I wondered if the problem was my language skills. I had never been tutored in the local dialect — even the Merina dialect of Malagasy was a challenge for me — and so I thought perhaps she did not understand that I only wanted her to work for a few minutes every day. A brilliant thought occurred to me.

"Come back tomorrow. My assistant, Degas, will be here, and he will explain to you in Malagasy. Maybe we can think of something." With that, she appeared happy, and departed.

I went to bed and slept soundly as the rats scurried over my head.

The next morning, just as the sun was rising, there was a terrible banging on my door. I opened it, and several people stormed in, screaming for Lalao. I could not make out anything they said except for the word *renirano*, which means river, and *lavo*, which means to fall, and so I thought perhaps Lalao had fallen in the river (just as I'd done the day before) and would be late coming to fix me breakfast. But it appeared they were looking for Lalao. I was completely bewildered, and couldn't understand a word.

"Lalao is not here," I explained, and before I could find out more about what was going on, they ran off.

I dressed and stepped outside, expecting more warm welcoming in what was now "my village."

Welcome Wagon wasn't exactly awaiting my appearance. Instead, right there, smack dab in front of my door, was a fire of twigs burning and smoking, with a big-bellied woman hanging upside down, smoking like a Virginia ham. Some young men were holding her by her feet, her long wet hair and limp arms dangling in the fire. With grave faces, several elder men and women were fanning the smoke in her face with banana fronds.

This was obviously weird. There was nothing at all about this in the ethnographies I'd read.

"Who is it?" I asked the eldest man standing near me. He, like many others, was scowling directly at me.

"It is the woman who came to you looking for work last night," he answered, "the one you would not hire." There was no mistaking that she was now dead.

I watched incredulously as they continued fanning her face with the smoke. And I thought about how badly I wanted to run in the house for my camera.

"What happened?" I finally asked.

"She went to the river behind your house, to bathe for her meeting with you," he explained, "and she fell in the river and drowned."

This was no way to get acquainted.

I continued to stand, silently, watching.

"*Fanafody!!!*" one of the elder women shouted, "We need *fanafody!!!*" They needed medicine. They were all looking at me. They knew that in with all that ridiculous *vazaha* stuff I'd brought, there must be a boxful of medicine.

The scowling man next to me said, "She needs *fanafody*. *Fodigasy* (Malagasy medicine, or plant medicine) is not strong enough. We need *vazaha* medicine."

What could I tell them? Our medicines *are* strong. But not strong enough for dead.

"*Tsy misy,*" (There isn't any), I explained, "There is no *vazaha* medicine for her. It is not that strong."

They stomped out the fire.

"Get your camera," the scowling man said, "take pictures for her family," and with that, he and the others motioned with their heads for me to hurry back in my house and get the camera. When I returned, they hoisted her on the shoulders of some strong young men, and motioned for me to follow.

Then the wailing began.

Nety was taken to her uncle's home (for I learned that she did not live in Ranotsara, but had only come to the village of her uncle when she learned there was potential work with a *vazaha*) and there the women undressed and cleaned her. She was then dressed in her best dress, her hair combed and pinned up, and she was wrapped in *lamba* (cloths). This done, she was taken to the *trano-be*, or "big house," a large one-room cement-floored house that I was to learn was used for funeral services, dances, celebrations, meetings, and ceremonies.

Young men from her family were sent to the forest where they selected a fine tree, chopped it down, stripped it of its bark, and brought it to the village. This done, it was hollowed out as a coffin, and Nety's *lamba*, by now dripping with bodily fluids, were changed. Wrapped in a white sheet, she was placed in the hollowed out tree, and visitation continued.

For three days and three nights, all non-essential work, including school and farming, stopped. People came from villages throughout the area to pay respects. Everyone was well dressed, and except for the wailing which never ceased inside the *trano-be*, the village took on a festive mood as people visited with cousins and friends, ate well, and drank *toaka gasy*. Everyone gave a gift, either money or food or *lamba*. The *trano-be* was always full, throughout the day and night. Nety was never left alone, and her mother never left her side, as she fanned the flies from her daughter's face for three days and three nights.

On the third day, a cow was sacrificed, its meat and organs distributed to everyone in the village. The village gathered, and her eldest maternal uncle, Koto, recited the *kabary*. The *kabary* is a late eighteenth-century speech form introduced during the rise of the Merina by Anrianampoinimerina to provide an oratorical means of recording—and creating—history (Bloch 1986; Larson1992). It now serves many purposes, including replicating ethnic identities (Larson 1992) and providing a means of social resistance through public speech (Hanson 1997). In this instance, the *kabary* served as a formalized means through which one could both honor the dead, establish the dead's ties to her lineage, and pressure the community to offer gifts to the family.

By reciting —in the text of the *kabary*—the name of each person who gave a gift, and the exact monetary amount or number of *lamba*, people knew who gave and who did not give, and were accordingly judged as to the appropriateness of the gift. Everyone was expected to give something, no matter how small, and to omit an offering would in this way bring public disgrace. Conversely, by making a generous offer, one aligned themselves with the family of the dead, thereby establishing the expectation of reciprocity. In so doing, however, they would either be expected to provide equally to others with subsequent deaths, or be judged as having acted prejudicially.

When the *kabary* was concluded, vines, which had been burning quietly throughout the speech, were removed from the smoldering ashes which had softened them, and wrapped around the coffin, then tightly tied to seal the lid closed. A few pieces of *kitay*, or wood fuel, were left to burn and tossed in with the grass mats which had lain under Nety's body. Along with the *lamba* she had worn, these objects were gathered together. The *kitay* and the *lamba* would keep her warm, while the smoldering flames and smoke would keep the *biby* [ghosts] away.

Nety's body was hoisted high and a procession followed it out of the village, as it passed over the head of the young toddling son her death had left orphaned. By passing over his head, she blessed and protected him for one last time. Her body was taken to the ancestral tomb of the Zafinaraina lineage, and the *lamba*, *kitay*, and grass mats were taken to a distant grove of trees for disposal.

With her body carried away, amidst the chanting and singing of French colonial military songs by the pall bearers, village life resumed.

In the year that followed, the death of Nety was explained in multiple ways. It confounded the villagers, because the river was not very deep. The spot where Nety fell was knee-deep with no current. And she was not found in the river, but laying dead on the bank.

My first thoughts, conditioned as they are by cheap novels, Hollywood, and lurid urban newspapers, ran toward homicide. But murder, while it happens, does not happen often enough in Madagascar that one would find themselves murdered by a competitor for the job of making a bed, or for very many other reasons.[1] As much as finding a woman drowned on a river bank next to a shallow river might sound suspicious

---

1. During my visits to Madagascar I only learned of three murders, all tied to the social changes of development and involving foreigners. The first, and most celebrated, was the murder of a young Malagasy man who had become so well-respected as a wildlife guide (including in Ranomafana) that the high wages and many gifts the *vazaha* bestowed on him were said to have contributed to his unexplained murder, believed to have been provoked by envy (see Quammen 1991). The second occurred during my stay in Madagascar, when a young female Peace Corps worker was sexually assaulted and murdered while jogging; while I do not know the details of this killing, it prompted much talk. Peace Corps workers I spoke to who knew both the victim and her alleged killer indicated that she had been telling women that they did not need to agree to unwanted sexual advances by this man. Whether or not there is any truth to this account I do not know, but the Peace Corps workers I spoke to interpreted her death as caution against introducing or advocating feminist perspectives (an irony given the outspoken nature of many Malagasy women, whom I found to be far more feminist than many "free" American women I know). They further indicated that this act was regarded as a consequence of white foreigners interfering in local lives. The third was a more typical tale of a European tourist who was said to be drunk and flashing his money; he was reportedly stabbed on a dark street as he tried to hail a cab back to his hotel. Since returning, I have learned of two other murders, both of research assistants employed to assist an American social scientist; they were alleged to have been murdered in retribution for their success at securing the positions.

to me, the truth was, murder was highly improbable. At least, murder by a mortal.

Nety had awoken at four or four thirty, a very early hour even by Malagasy standards, and gone to the river to bathe. It was still dark, and so the *biby* (water spirits, nature spirits), were out. Everyone knew that it was dangerous to go to the river at that hour.

Some consequently attributed her death to the *biby*.

As the months unfolded, however, other explanations were whispered. Nety was found with blood between her legs. Perhaps she had been trying to perform an abortion? Many people concluded that the reason Nety died was because she had tried to abort her baby, and the ancestors struck her dead for the offense.

But several months later, when I discussed the incident with the RNPP physician, he remembered her. He had been treating her for epilepsy. She had no income, and could no longer afford the medicine. In all likelihood, he explained, she had a seizure in the river, and in her seizure, had somehow managed to reach the riverbank.

"And that would explain the blood between her legs," I surmised, "because she was miscarrying perhaps?"

I raised my theory with various people in the village. It seemed likely, all agreed. But still, the *biby* were angry.

"But would she have died, do you think, if she'd had the medicine to stop the seizures?" I asked Nirina, who sat behind my house looking out to the river where Nety's spirit now resided.

"Oh, if she had the *fanafody* for the seizures, then she would be alive. Seizures are very powerful," Nirina explained, demonstrating with a feigned seizure that rattled her whole aged skeleton. "Without medicine, many Tanala die from them. She needed *fanafody*, and the *fanafody gasy* is not strong. But now we must pay for *fanafody vazaha* [Western medicines], and they are very expensive. She could not pay for the medicine. If she had had the medicine, the *biby* might have frightened her, but they would not have killed her. *Fanafody gasy* would have cured her."

"What *fanafody gasy*?" I asked, "How would it have cured her?"

"*Apanga*," Nirina answered, "the plant used to bring back the soul. It is used to treat unconsciousness. The plant is burned and the smoke inhaled. You saw how we tried to bring back her soul by burning the *apanga*." I recalled the way Nety hung over the burning vines, with the banana fronds fanning the smoke into her face, and the frantic elders calling for stronger medicine, *vazaha* medicine.

Nirina ended her explanation with another feigned seizure and a loud laugh at her own performance.

After reflecting on her comments, I later asked her what she meant by Tanala dying. Was she suggesting that Betsileo do not need the same medicines as Tanala, that Tanala are more susceptible to death than Betsileo?

Nirina sighed and gave me a long and patient look. *"Ho maty Betsileo, ho maty Tanala, ho maty Vazaha! Maty daholo,"* she declared with good humor, perhaps wondering if I realized my own mortality. ["The Betsileo will die, the Tanala will die, you foreigners will die! Everyone dies."]

"We are the Tanala. Everyone here is Tanala. People who live here are no different from Betsileo, but Betsileo live near Fianarantsoa. They have hospitals there, they do not have the *tavy* fields we have here. We live in the forest. If they come here, then they live the lives of Tanala. Then they will have our sickness and die along with us."

I continued to ponder the many explanations for Nety's death that were whispered about the village. No patterns emerged initially, but with time and many repetitions, it appeared that while the older people focused on her need for medicine for her seizures, younger women (and some young adult men I was told by my male informant) were more convinced she had been punished for her alleged sin of trying to abort, a rumor for which there was no evidence. While it is entirely possible that older people wondered the same thing, they may have been less willing to discuss the topic with me, particularly those who were Catholic. I wondered, as well, if the difference in explanations could be attributed to older people having more experience with seizures as something treatable by medicine, and younger people knew only of a seizure as something uncontrollable. I will never know. The subject of Nety's death was off-limits for structured interviews. It lived on in rumor only.

With the burial of Nety, I thought I would see no more sudden death, and wondered how I would go about learning about how people treated sickness. I soon discovered, however, that death and sickness were daily events, and watched awkwardly and horrified as child after child, adult after adult, fell ill and died.

A Quest for Diagnosis

Shortly after my arrival in the village, and as I noted one death after another, I urgently appealed to project management to send the traveling physician to the village. As Ranotsara had not officially been removed from the list of target villages, and the absence of health care for the last three years remained unexplained officially, I felt it was appropriate for me to raise my concerns about village health status to the project physician, Dr. Tovo. Dr. Tovo is a young, well-educated physician with considerable concern for the health of the rural poor, and much pride in his education in tropical medicine. Working long hours away from his family, he would travel great distances, hiking over treacherous terrain with a backpack full of his few medicines and medical supplies, to check on a broken bone, or follow-up on the care of an ailing patient. He was the sole physician for the estimated 30,000 residents of the Ranomafana National Park peripheral zone, and worked only with the assistance of two nurses and one "midwife," untrained in midwifery, but whose responsibility it was to dispense birth control pills.[2] He reported making approximately 1,000,000 fmg ($250) per month, receiving a monthly raise of approximately 10,000 fmg ($2.50) after two years with the project.

Upon hearing of the deaths and the spreading illnesses of the village, Dr. Tovo felt that visiting the village should be a priority. Moreover, my research on health and access to medicines in the region suggested to him opportunities for collaboration in which we could share knowledge. Consequently, within a month of my arrival in Ranotsara, the residents received their first health team visit in over three years.[3] Dr. Tovo later informed me that the health of the village was perhaps the worst he had seen in the entire region. He reasoned that the wet and humid environment, characterized by irrigated rice fields surrounding the entire village and creating a miniature island on which the village rested, compounded by poor sanitation, poor water quality, its distance from the main road, ex-

---

2. In contrast, one physician and one nurse were hired shortly before my arrival to treat the project staff.

3. Oddly, on the day of his arrival, I received an unexpected summons to appear that same day in distant Ifanadiana, to provide evidence I had paid for my visa (seven months after arriving in Madagascar). As such, I was unable to attend the visit by the traveling health team, and upon inquiring of the nurse if I might discuss the visit, was informed that he had been instructed by the American Project Director not to speak with me. Fortunately, I was able to examine records of the visit provided to me by another, and after interviewing residents, learned of the events of the day. Dr. Tovo himself indicated that his decision to visit the village was regarded with surprising suspicion by project administrators, who questioned him at length about his interest in the village. He said that he had never before been questioned about a village he attended. At the same time that project administration expressed such concern for the doctor's work, however, I was struck by an equally surprising lack of concern for the residents. Indeed, during a visit to the home of project manager one evening, she rhetorically asked me, as she stirred some cooking on the stove, how things were going in the village. I responded that another child had died. Her reply was a mumbled, "humph," prompting me to add, "that's the eleventh so far." She looked directly at me and announced, "I think this gravy needs more salt." One can only speculate as to her response had I pointed out eleven lemurs had dropped dead. Nonetheless, Dr. Tovo was instructed that he was not to return to the village and it was not until the day after my scheduled departure, that project administrators directed him to return.

treme poverty of its residents, and poor education about health matters, all contributed to the sickness that prevailed. Among the illnesses that struck him were widespread scabies (often infected), infected circumcisions, parasites, and respiratory disorders. Of the 39 people he saw that day, 10 were treated for intestinal parasites, 14 for scabies (including five people with infected scabies), and 16 for respiratory infections.[4] Perhaps the most severe of this latter category was that suffered by Lanto.

Lanto was a bit of an outcast in Ranotsara. Her hair grew wild and she left it uncombed; she kept to herself and rarely joined group activities. The death of her first husband, clearly by *mpamosavy* [witches], as *toaka* is known only to kill when a *mpamosavy* poisons it, brought lingering gossip as to who killed him and why. Although she was the granddaughter of one of the village founders and the sister of the *mpanjaka*, her status as a Zafindraraoto, accompanied by her poverty and social seclusion, cast her as an outsider in her own village.

Lanto describes herself as a *mpamboly*, or farmer, and proudly proclaims that she was born and raised in Ranotsara. When asked her ethnicity she says that she is "Betsileo," because her ancestors were "Betsileo," an identification that cannot be regarded too rigidly, as ethnic identity was constantly shifting. She also indicates that she was once a Catholic, but no longer practices because she is not interested in attending services or praying. She has had two years of schooling and can neither read nor write. After the death of her first husband, she remarried, but her second husband, whom she described as having "a different head," than hers, moved away nearly two years earlier, leaving her to raise their five children on her own, including two young and underfed toddlers.[5] With limited land of her own, Lanto struggled to feed and clothe her children, but a cyclone the previous year had wiped out her crops, and so, she reported, she sold her banana trees (which she estimated to be about 100 in number) to Rivo for 10,000 fmg (about $2.50). She was left with *tavy*, but no one to farm it. Her eldest son had moved to Tulear and she had not seen him since. Another son had gone to live with Pascal, when Lanto could no longer afford to feed him; in exchange for room and board, he worked Pascal's fields, leaving no one to help Lanto farm her land.

Her own health was poor—bone thin and slow moving, she looked much older than a woman in her early or mid-forties, and a chronic bloody

---

4. These numbers cannot be taken to represent the health status of the village as a whole, but reflect only those who were in the village at the time of his visit, had cash available to purchase medicines, and chose to see the doctor.

5. Only her eldest daughter has had any schooling, of about five years.

cough limited her strength. When strong enough, she worked for Rivo, Philippe, or Pascal for food and cash, receiving about 1,000 fmg (about 25 cents at the time of my stay, and about two-thirds the going rate) and one kapoaka[6] of rice (valued at about 1,500 fmg at the time of my interview).

Her economic strategies were, during the time I knew her, mixed and limited. She told me that she would not borrow money because she could not repay it. She said that she worked a few days a week, but in truth, she probably worked less than that. "*Mitady any sakafo*," she would say, "I look for food." From what I saw, and what was told to me by herself and others, Lanto and her children ate and consumed very little, having meals twice a day. Her meals consisted of rice and greens, and sometimes wild forest or sweet potatoes. Like many in Ranotsara, she often lacked rice, so she and her children often ate tubers.

Lanto was among the many women who met with me on several occasions for long and personal interviews, often lasting half the day. Her constant phlegm-filled coughing concerned me, and I asked how long she had been coughing so. Since the birth of her last child, she disclosed, she had been suffering from *marikoditra* [a fever with chills] and the *kohaka* [cough]. She did not know the cause, she said, but believed it came from working in the fields during the time of her pregnancy and following the birth of her child. It was then, she said, that she first became so very tired and her illness began. The illness started with dizziness and vomiting, she soon became weak and had trouble walking. She had a constant headache, and no appetite. The illness, she said, has made it difficult to work. Now, three years later, it had moved to her chest. Regarding it as life-threatening, she was even more concerned with her failing eyesight. But no one in the village had eye glasses, nor the means to obtain them. The closest optometry was in Fianarantsoa, a full-day's voyage and with the cost of the *taxi-brousse*[7], food, and lodging, not to mention the optometrist's fee and the glasses themselves, beyond Lanto's, and everyone else's, means.

And so she had grown accustomed to her failing eyesight in the same way that she had grown accustomed to her cough. She would take "red pills" [antibiotics] and aspirin periodically, she said, whenever the traveling physician visited; she had not had them since he stopped coming, she reported.[8]

---

6. A kapoaka is a Nestle milk can full, usually of rice, and is a standard unit of measurement.

7. A *taxi-brousse* is a public "taxi," usually an old battered station wagon or smaller car, in which up to 14 people might squeeze.

8. While Lanto indicated her illness began two or three years prior, her disclosure that she had been taking medicine for the pills during the period when the first traveling physician, prior to Dr. Tovo, had visited monthly, suggests that either the illness was of much longer duration, or she was taking the pills for something else.

She said that she refused to take *fanafody gasy*, claiming it did not help her. "Only the doctor's medicines have helped," she insisted, adding that she paid 1,250 fmg for each injection the previous doctor gave her.

Contrary to her claim that she did not use *fanafody gasy*, she did tell me that she went to an *ombiasa* two years prior, to treat her illness. Rakoto told her that she was suffering from *bilo* [known locally as ghost sickness; in other parts of the island it refers to a type of possession]. To treat her, she said that he played the *kabosy* [home crafted string instrument] to find the *bilo*, but he did not find it. She paid him 3,500 fmg and two liters of *toaka* for his services. He gave her some dried leaves, she said, but she could not recall, or would not reveal, the names of the leaves. She drank teas made from the leaves, and inhaled the steam from the brewing leaves for a week.

"I stopped," she said, "I did not believe it was *bilo*. It was from having a baby, or maybe from working too hard," she considered. As I inquired further, she explained, "This illness comes with being tired from giving birth; women get it when they have children. But maybe I just worked too hard and got tired." Lanto added that she did not believe having children was a health problem, as I had inquired in previous interviews. "The sicknesses of women," she told me, "are sick backs. Our work is hard, and it hurts our backs."

Her comment corresponds to Avotri and Walters' (1999) finding that women in the Volta region of Ghana, West Africa were not as concerned about reproductive health as they were about health problems related to their work, including "worrying too much," having difficulty sleeping, chronic tiredness, headaches, and bodily aches.

> Women talked about the medication they took for various ailments, their visits to pharmacies, health centers and hospitals, as well as the prohibitive cost of these, and a handful of women spoke in terms of their responsibility for their health. But these were by no means the main emphasis in the interviews. Instead, women talked about the ways in which their day-to-day lives created or exacerbated the health problems they experienced. One particularly strong emphasis was on the ways in which women's work influences their health (Avotri and Walters 1999:1124).

Lanto's understanding that her illness was likely to be related to the circumstances of her life, rather than possession by a *bilo*, suggested an astute comprehension of the social factors shaping health in the tropical forest. But the *increase* in illness, she felt, was related to the cold weather. The cold brought on the back aches and neck aches that plagued so many adult women, she suggested, while the coughing that was common to all children was likewise an illness of the weather. "But the poor," she said, in almost a whisper, "get all illnesses."

Unhappy with the treatment Rakoto had prescribed, because, she explained, it did not cure her, she did not return. Nonetheless, she remained hopeful, if not confident, that Rakoto could cure other illnesses. Doctors, she revealed, cure illnesses of the body, but *ombiasa* cure illnesses of the spirit. Fearing her children had such an illness, when they began having headaches and coughing severely and constantly, she sent each of them to Rakoto. Just as he did with her, Rakoto gave the children plants for drinking and inhalation, but they were not the same plants he had given her, and he guarded the names of the plants so she was unable to tell me what they were. But the children did not get better. One child became unconscious and Rakoto did nothing, she recalled, with a trace of anger. Fortunately, her brother pointed out to her that the child was very hot and instructed her to cool him with cold water. She did so, and he recovered. She recalled with despair how the children were cured on their own, not by Rakoto, she stressed. Nonetheless, she paid him 175 fmg for his services.

Lanto's quest for treatment of her chronic cough and difficulty breathing, did not stop with Rakoto. She recalled going to Ranomafana shortly afterwards, where she was told she needed an injection. She said she was not told the name of the illness or the medicine, but recalled the price of 1,250 fmg quite clearly.

"The injections made me better, like the red pills. But I didn't have the money to keep getting them, and the trip was very long. So the cough would come back."

"Did you use plant medicines?" I asked, for the third or fourth time, broaching the question from multiple directions to see if I could stumble upon some undisclosed secret of the local botany.

"*Ahibalala*," she answered, matter-of-factly, as she had each time before. Like so many others, she turned to *ahibalala* the way an American turns to Tylenol or Echinacea root. The only other medicines she admitted to using were those she used to maintain her teeth, a method she learned from her father.

I asked Lanto if knowing more about the plants would help the health of the people living in Ranotsara. "No," she said, "we get sick more often than you *vazaha* because we do not have *fanafody*. What we need is more *fanafody vazaha*, not more plants. But there is no money for them."

Lanto, having exhausted herself talking to me about things she found to be so obvious, was among the first to visit Dr. Tovo when he came to the village. Because his visit was unannounced, most adults were working their fields when he arrived; many of those working *tavy* fields missed the visit altogether, remaining unaware that health care had come to the village until it had once again gone. But because Lanto's health was so poor, she worked little. As such, she was at home, cooking for her children, when the doctor arrived. After waiting her turn outside the makeshift clinic set up in the *trano-be* ["big house" used for ceremonies and funerals], she timidly approached the young, educated doctor, and asked him for help.

Listening to her lungs through his stethoscope, watching her cough with every effort to speak, and questioning her about the course and symptoms of her illness, he became concerned that she might have tuberculosis, a fairly common illness he encountered as he hiked from village to village. Knowing how contagious and severe such an illness is, he prescribed Tetracycline and Chloroquine (for a fever that accompanied her cough) and advised her to go as soon as possible to the clinic in Ranomafana. To be sure she did so, when meeting my assistant in the town of Ranomafana a few days later, Dr. Tovo shared his concerns and asked that I encourage her to go.

My verbal encouragement was not necessary, however, and Lanto went obligingly to the clinic, without feeling the need to check in with the *vazaha* about what she should do. She walked the 7 km distance in the rain, taking a day off work and leaving her children in the care of the eldest. Upon arriving, she found the clinic was closed with no reason stated. She returned to Ranotsara promptly, reaching the village by the end of the day.

She shared her frustration with me. "It is always this way, I am not surprised. Sometimes they are open and sometimes they are not. I walked all that way and back again, for nothing!"

This time, I did encourage her to return. But she expressed her concerns with me that she wouldn't have the money for the supplies, such as alcohol or cotton, or for a blood test, which she anticipated. Her concern was well founded; while treatment was free, supplies were not. Moreover, she would need to eat. I advanced her the money for supplies, and my assistant, Degas, made an appointment for her for the following Friday.

So once again, she left her children and hiked the 7km to town. This time the clinic was open and a nurse drew her blood, and told her to return the following Monday. Hiking back again, she returned to the village by nightfall, completely exhausted. She made no mention of the trip to me, and made it clear that she was too tired to talk about it. On the following Monday, and without comment, she returned for the third time. Once there, after waiting hours to be seen, they drew her blood again. She neither asked, nor did they explain, why they were repeating the test. The blood drawn, she was told to return the next day. Weakened and hungry, she tried to visit her family in Ranomafana for some rest and a meal, but they were not there. She returned to Ranotsara without having eaten all day.

On Tuesday she returned to Ranomafana for the fourth time. This time, she was told to return the following day with a vial of her sputum, which inexplicably, they would not accept at that time. She said she was too worn out from all the hiking and would wait until Friday to return. But by the time Friday came, Lanto was fed up. She refused to return, having made four round-trip hikes over the mountainous terrain with a burning fever and severe respiratory problems.[9]

Degas, my assistant, followed up with the clinic to find out if she did indeed have tuberculosis. The findings were negative, but there was no attempt made by the clinicians to find out what was wrong with her. She was simply sick, with *kohaka*.

Lanto concluded that the antibiotics were all she had needed in the first place and the cough would plague her for the rest of her life. "I can drink *ahibalala* when it is bad," she concluded.

Under the Skin: Suffering with Scabies

Scabies is a highly-contagious and absolutely miserable affliction. Caused by a microscopic insect that burrows under the skin, it produces extreme and unrelenting itching. The pharmaceutical treatment is to wash all clothes, towels, and bedding with a pesticide-based lotion (Benzyl benzoate) marketed as Ascabial and available only through a physician's prescription. This lotion is also applied liberally to all infected areas of the skin.

There is no plant or other organic substance known to the residents of Ranotsara which will relieve the pain or cure the condition as effectively. Cleanliness is regarded, by Malagasy and Western health professionals alike, as the most important prophylactic treatment, but the highly contagious nature of scabies makes even thorough and repeated scrubbing with soap, even if available, no guarantee that it will not spread.

My fieldwork began, after public introductions and Nety's fatal seizure, with door-to-door introductions. Accompanied by Degas, notebook in hand and an explanatory speech of my research objectives memorized, I visited each family and interrogated them with invasive but excessively polite demographic questions.

---

9. Farmer (1999) discusses the difficulty rural peasants face when trying to access diagnostic tests and treatment for tuberculosis, thereby contributing to its rapid spread among the poor. He points out that rather than being a problem of "patient non-compliance," (Farmer 1999:212) the high rate of death from tuberculosis, a disease which is curable but continues to kill millions of people each year, is related to structural inequalities that enable certain groups of people to live in healthier environments and have access to early diagnosis and effective treatment, while other groups of people are forced to live in crowded environments with little or no access to the early intervention and effective drugs that would cure their disease.

Kala's husband, Zanabelo, was of the Zafinaraina lineage. His mother, Bodo, was the daughter of Raminstiry, who had married the alleged *andevo*, Ikalahafa. As such, although he had retained the well-respected lineage through his mother's paternity, it was tainted with his grandfather's intermarriage of caste. As I have previously indicated, such intermarriage does not necessarily render one impoverished; indeed, the wealthiest individuals in the village, who control most of the land and resources, were themselves descended from this alliance. Consequently, Zanabelo's ancestry alone did not account for the extreme poverty in which he and his family lived.

Zanabelo was relatively land-rich, but lacked the labor to farm his land, which included irrigated rice fields, *tavy*, and cash crops. In addition to the rice grown in the irrigated and swidden fields, he intercropped his *tavy* fields with lentils, manioc and beans. His cash crops included sugar cane, bananas, manioc and coffee, and he raised chickens for food and trade.

Zanabelo explained that when his father was younger, they worked the land together, and crops were abundant. But as his father aged and weakened, it was left to Zanabelo alone to work the fields, along with his wife. He occasionally received help from his family, but in recent years, his cousins Rivo, Philippe and Pascal, had prospered and were hence preoccupied with their own lands; his other cousins were working for them for wages that Zanabelo could not match.

His needs had increased in recent years as well. Working his fields alone has required better tools, such as shovels and knives, and as his family grew at the same time that he lost the help of his family in farming his land, the rice that he and his wife were able to grow on their own declined. As such, he has been forced to buy rice at market, along with sugar, coffee[10], petrol, salt, *lamba* (for funeral offerings) and clothes. When he has the money, he'll buy a bit of meat for his family. Otherwise, they get by on the rice, beans, greens and manioc they grow.

Kala and Zanabelo were among the few villagers who consistently reported that they regarded themselves as "Betsileo." (In contrast, Zanabelo's wealthier brother, Raboly, consistently reported that he considered himself "Tanala.") Married twenty years, they had three surviving children, at the time of my fieldwork, 16 year-old Claude, 7 year-old Tonga, and 2 year-old Ravo. Five of their children had died, the last, a twelve-year old son who had been schooled "for many years," died suddenly the

---

10. A small cache of coffee is considered relatively essential, in that it is offered to honored visitors, as well as used as a medicine to treat *tazo* [fevers]. Its bitter taste is believed to be medicinal. Coffee as a daily beverage, however, is rare because it is too costly, both in the loss of its sale, and in the fuel wood necessary to roast it and the time needed to roast and pound it.

previous year, after complaining of a headache and lying down to sleep. He never awoke. Zanabelo himself had only five or six years of school; he can read and write a bit, "*fa tsy tsara*" [but not well].

Zanabelo explained that he often needs to borrow money from his cousins to make it through the year. If he is able, he says, he would repay as soon as possible. If not, he is forced to wait for the following year's crops, at which time he repays, whether in cash or in rice, twice the amount he has borrowed. If he could not repay the loan, he said, his cousins would take his land [I could not ascertain whether or not this was true, although it was repeated by others.].

Zanabelo regarded the relationship between food and health as simple. You have to eat well to be healthy. But in regard to the most serious health problems he perceived, he indicated that *hantana*, or scabies, was one of the worst, yet unrelated to food. His wife, Kala, in contrast, did not regard *hantana* as a significant health problem.

Kala is an illiterate woman in her late 30s who had lived in Ranotsara for nineteen years. She has never gone to school and, like her husband, does not practice or profess Catholicism. Kala is very shy, but with a warm personality that slowly unfolds. She is openly devoted to her children, and rocks her youngest in her arms as we speak.

They are covered with scabies, so badly infected that the two-year old looks like a burn victim, and 7 year-old Tonga digs at his legs furiously while we talk, smiling broadly all the time. Tonga's smile is so constant, in fact, that in nearly all of my photos of children crowded together for a photo opportunity, it is Tonga whose face is always the most noticeable, his smile so outstanding. As he scratches and digs deeply into his scabies-scarred legs, he appears unaware of the pain. His mother, as well, scratches unconsciously at her hands and her feet, the red-dotted rash visible between her fingers and toes.

"*Hantana* is not one of our problems," she tells me, in answer to my many questions of health and living conditions. "We have it all the time. We learn to suffer with it. *Sempotra* [respiratory problems] and *tazo* [fevers] are problems."

Despite her repeated comments that she ignored *hantana* and did nothing to treat it, she later admitted that she used a medicine made from *volopotsy* leaves, found in the *hibo-hibo* [*tavy* regrowth]. "Everybody uses it; everybody knows where to get it."

But this comment, too, brought with it contradictory testimony, as she told me that the plant had become increasingly difficult to find with the spread of *tavy*, and later remarked that it could be found everywhere and was in no short supply. Moreover, she twice told me that she did not know of the plant until she moved to Ranotsara, and learned of it from the other women, while one other time she said that she had learned of it from her father. Rather than dismissing her comments as irrelevant, I was intrigued by them, because since Ranotsara is a patrilocal community, I found it fairly common for women to remark that they learned of new medicines upon moving to Ranotsara. While they may have learned of these medicines from other women, in many cases this knowledge had been transmitted through males. As such, contrary to other findings in Madagascar that women are the primary keepers of indigenous knowledge of plant medicines (Sussman 1988), I found that this was not always true. Women's roles in finding and dispensing the medicines were often central, but men's roles were also significant in transmitting knowledge of plant medicines, as will be discussed further.

Whether or not Kala had learned of *volopotsy* as an indigenous medicine for *hantana* from her parents, and brought the knowledge with her, or learned of it after arriving in Ranotsara, I do not know. But she did explain that she had been using it daily on herself and all of her children for the last six months and they seemed to be improving.

"It doesn't look like it's working," I subjectively replied.

"It takes a very long time," she admitted.

I suggested she use Ascabiol and gave her a supply, explaining how to use it and warning her of its toxicity. I emphasized that she should not let any of it get into open sores. Knowing that I was, once again, interfering with the objectivity of the research process, I felt it would be unprincipled to leave the children with such a painful condition that would only worsen when I had a medicine I knew would be effective.

Shortly after this visit, Dr. Tovo came to Ranotsara but Kala did not bring her children to him, later explaining to me that she lacked the money for the medicines he would prescribe and dispense.[11]

We met a few weeks later in my home. Kala had agreed to participate in a lengthy interview regarding women's health concerns and beliefs. Tonga played outside with some other boys. As we talked, we watched as he kicked a grapefruit around like a small soccer ball. The backs of his legs were charred black like his sister, and so severely infected that the blackened skin was split open with large wounds oozing white and yellow pus, but the injuries did not slow his movements, which were quick and lively.

"Are there any health problems in your family, right now?" I asked.

"No, *salama tsara izahay*," she answered [we are all healthy].

"What about the *hantana*?" I prompted.

"*Sitrana tsara*" [it is all (well) cured], she replied.

"Did you use the medicine I gave you?"

---

11. There would have been a modest fee charged for the medicines, but in hardship cases where medicine was needed, Dr. Tovo often waived the fee.

"Yes, it is all gone, thank you."

Degas, my assistant, interrupted in English. "I have to ask her about his legs. They are very infected." I told him to go ahead.

"*Hadiniko!*" [I forgot!] she replied, suppressing a giggle. Yes, she agreed, his legs were quite bad. He had been tending cattle in the woods for Rivo, she explained, and came back itching. He must have rubbed his legs against some type of plant that caused the itching.

I asked if we could look at Tonga's legs. She called him in, and on closer examination, it was clear his wounds were very infected. They smelled foul and the ulcers had burrowed deep into his flesh, reaching as high as his buttocks. The lymph glands in his groin were swollen the size of small eggs. I urged her to get him to the clinic in Ranomafana for treatment. She answered that she would wait, and when her husband returned from *an-tsaha*, ask him. I also noticed that Tonga was wearing a new necklace, with a piece of wood and a plastic bead tied around a length of string. I asked what it was.

"*Ody katry*," she answered, proud to show she me she had, in fact, done something to safeguard her son's health, despite what I might have thought of his legs.

Katry is an indigenous diagnostic category for fevers and seizures that affect small children. To prevent *katry*, Zanabelo's cousin, Alarobia, an *ombiasa* and *mpanjaka* who lives in the neighboring village of Ambato-vory, prepares amulets for all the local children to wear around their necks. At the time of my fieldwork, he charged 350 fmg (about 10 cents, U.S.) for the *ody katry*, and nearly all the children in the nearby villages wore them.

After she left I asked Degas and Lalao if it was common for a woman to ask her husband permission to get medical treatment for a child. Both immediately corrected me. Kala did not need to ask his permission for medical care, but it would be up to Zanabelo to carry Tonga across the mountains. As such, unless it was such an emergency that another male in the community would undertake the endeavor, Kala was acting appropriately by awaiting her husband's return and consulting him.

That evening, he came to my home and asked my opinion of his son's legs. Were they really that bad?, he asked, weighing whether or not he should leave his fields idle to take his son to Ranomafana. I assured him that I was no doctor, but I was very concerned about the infection in Tonga's legs. I urged him to get him to the doctor as soon as possible, and in the meantime, keep the legs clean and free of dirt. I gave him soap and clean bandages. He thanked me, and the next morning, carried Tonga over the mountains to Ranomafana.

He returned at nightfall, but the parents did not appear to be keeping the wounds clean. The clinic nurse, Robert, who had treated Tonga in Ranomafana, chastised the mother for washing his wounds. He explained that she had probably broken the skin open by repeated washing. Robert gave Tonga an injection of antibiotics and nothing else. Tonga's legs were as dirty when he returned as when he left. The parents concluded that there was nothing wrong with their son and I had overreacted. For the first day after their return, they tied the bandages around his legs, but removed them when they became dirty. Tonga's legs did heal slowly, while the scabies continued to rage through the community, and the babies and children appeared to barely notice.

I was not alone in my perplexity at the manner in which an illness that is so miserable to live with would remain minimally treated or even completely neglected. Many of the older residents expressed disapproval at what they described as the laziness of the younger generation. The use of the word *kamo* [lazy] to describe young adults who labor strenuously twelve hours a day, seven days a week, struck me as paradoxical when uttered by local elders (while I found the same adjective, when used by sedentary project personnel and other *vazaha*, as it frequently was, to be plainly racist). Some older people attributed the *hantana* pandemic to the dirtiness [*maloto*] of the village area, the lack of soap and the lack of money to purchase it, and a lack of attention to personal cleanliness. One person who claimed to have no explanation for why the illness was so neglected was the *ombiasa*, Naina.

"Curing *hantana* is not hard," he said, "if it is caught early. But it is difficult to cure when it becomes serious." Naina listed the many medicines he used to treat skin disorders, only one of which he finds in the forest.

"*Kimboinbohy*, I find in the *savoka* [regrowth], *tainguaka* is a moss. It works well. I find it in the forest sometimes, growing on dead trees, but it is also in the *savoka* [secondary growth, following burning of *tavy*]. *Sevatrandraka*, *tanamangamay*." He counted them on his fingers, looking out the window to the forest in the distance. "*Tanamangamay* is found along the road. And *kitsiotsiona* is another good medicine. It grows everywhere. The medicines for *hantana* are easy to find. But they only work if it is caught early."

"Why isn't it caught early?" I asked him.

"*Tsy fantatro* [I don't know]," he answered, "There have only been two people to come to me to be cured of *hantana*. One from here, and my wife, before she died. I cured them both. But others do not come. And now the *hantana* is everywhere, like venereal disease[12]."

---

12. Naina's remark was revealing, but I did not have any evidence of venereal disease as a major health problem. Dr. Tovo diagnosed one person with a venereal disease during the period of my fieldwork, and in discussions with residents it was believed that it was usually an illness of men, and unless a woman has symptoms, residents believe that she does not need treatment. Due to the sensitive nature of the question, I did not pursue much inquiry into people's experience with venereal diseases. As for AIDS, there was an

172 · Endangered Species

Naina indicated that he did not know why people would not come to him for treatment of *hantana*. He did not think that they went to the *vazaha* doctor either, he told me. "They ignore it," he concluded. "I can't force them to come to me. And they don't use their own medicines, either. Not many people know the medicines to cure *hantana*. We have always had the illness, but not like now. I don't think many people know the medicines because it was never as common in the past, as it is now. They didn't need to know. Maybe they don't need to know now, either, if they can get the *dokotera*'s [doctor's] medicine. It works faster than mine. But it is expensive, so they wait until it is grave."

"Why do you think it is more common now?" I inquired, returning to his previous point.

"I don't know. I don't know what causes it. It is a malady of the skin. People get it from others who have it. *Toaka* [rum] and *sakay* [chile peppers] make it worse. They make it spread. If a person avoids these things, it is easier to cure. It's a good idea to wash if the *hantana* is moist. We have always had it. Now it is very bad, but even if people used my medicines or the *dokotera*'s medicine, we would still have it, but it would not be the same." Naina paused to drink some tea. He was silent for several awkward moments, before he looked up from his tea with a smile.

"The name has changed! Write this down. *Kidea* was the name of scabies in the past, and then it became *farasisa*[13], but when it started spreading, people could get it just by sitting in the same chair. If you touch someone with *hantana* now, and the liquid from it touches you, you will get it. Soon the whole village got it. That was about ten years ago. That was when the name was changed to *hantana*! I don't know why." He returned to concentrating on his tea, and I diligently wrote down his words.

Why scabies is so prevalent and why it remains untreated remains unclear. But it was clear that I did not notice older people with the disorder, yet infants were certain to get it within two weeks of their birth, and young adults were equally susceptible. Naina's children, however, did not have it.

---

awareness of SIDA (the French acronym for the disease) by all, and even one person remarked that it was an example of how the illnesses brought by *vazaha* kill faster than the illnesses spread from Malagasy to Malagasy. Surprisingly, however, AIDS has not spread as rapidly in Madagascar as it has in other parts of Africa, and at the time of my departure appeared to be largely concentrated in the port towns and the capital city. How quickly the disease will spread from these urban sites to rural areas is difficult to predict.

13. *Farasisa* has been frequently recorded in colonial and pre-colonial accounts of health conditions on the island to refer to a wide-range of subcutaneous skin disorders.

Parasites and Rice Fields

One evening in January, after a day spent visiting sick children, discussing medicines with their parents, and dispensing Nivaquine and aspirin to those with high fevers, there was a familiar knock at the door. It was twelve-year-old Toky's friendly nighttime visit, which had become a tradition of English and Malagasy greetings and riddles, Toky's infamous story-telling marathons, and his delivery of all the rumors I was not supposed to be hearing.

This time, however, I was surprised by the visit, because when I'd seen Toky earlier in the day, he was curled up on a corner of the dirt floor in his home, his head burning with fever and his mother feeding him soupy rice between his coughing. I opened the door to find him wrapped tightly in a dirty ragged blanket, the tears falling like rainfall from a face that until that day was perpetually beaming with humor and life.

"Janezi," he cried, "I am getting better since you came. My mother gave me *fanafody gasy*. It was *ahibalala*. Here," he said, offering me a torn slip of paper with the words *ahibalala aminy sempotra* [ahibalala for coughing] written carefully in ballpoint ink. "I already wrote it down for you so you can just put this in your notebook, and write, 'Toky's medicine'." He proudly smiled through his tears.

"Toky, you are so sick, you should be home sleeping. Come in, it's cold out there."

He came into the room and, as always, looked all around for signs of anything new. Noting some chocolate on the bedside table, he glanced at me with a teasing smile on his pale wet face.

"Here, Toky, I think you need some chocolate." I gave him a piece as he said, "Thank you," in crisp accented English. Happy, but still wrapped tightly in his blanket, he sat back in the comfortable wooden chair I'd had hauled liked a colonialist halfway across the island, and savored the chocolate in teeny bites. When he had finished, he took a deep breath and made his announcement.

"Janezi," he said, "I am afraid I am going to die, just like all my friends."

There was a strong melodrama to his words, but the truth they spoke could not be easily dismissed. The truth was, in a lifetime that wasn't much longer than my graduate studies, many of his friends had died, of malaria, respiratory problems, unexplained sudden illnesses. Today, with nearly every child sick inside his or her house and their parents staying home to tend them, the threat of death to more children was very real and in everyone's minds. Two important elders had died in the last six weeks; both had been strong and seemingly healthy. And three weeks prior, six year old Tsaralahy had died of malaria. Three more children would die within the month, with many more to follow. So while I had the sense that Toky's mother had sent him to play upon my sympathies and perhaps get cash or medicines or food, I also knew that what he spoke rang true. Toky might well be next, just as anyone could follow.

"Toky, you will not die," I insisted, "you are too smart for the *bilo* to catch you, and no one will let you die. We need you to keep us laughing!" I tried my best to cheer him up, but I have never been very good at that sort of thing. I knew he was in no mood for lies.

"I am afraid I have too many worms," he said, patting his swollen belly. It was true, Toky's belly was as bloated as a pregnant woman in her last trimester. There was no doubting that he had a belly full of worms.

"This morning I counted iPaul's worms. There were sixteen! Last week there were only seven!" Ever since learning, from the traveling health team, that they counted worms in stools, he had set out to monitor his little brother's health. Toky doted on his little brother as his greatest pride and happiness in life.

"I could not count all the worms *I* had, there were so many!"

"Yes, you do have many worms, and I can give you medicine for that, but they will come back. The whole village has worms."

Toky knew this. Everyone knew this. Worms were not something they believed were natural, but suffering with them had become natural. Everyone I spoke to in my interviews and informally, knew how it was that worms entered the body. The health team had told them, and they saw for themselves the worms swarming in the irrigated rice fields.

I was stunned, myself, when I first trudged out to Philippe's rice fields to join the women he'd hired to plant rice, and took a look at the water. As elderly Nirina and young Colette both moved aside to make a place for me between them, I scooped up a batch of rice shoots, and shoved the clumps of muddied roots into the warm brown water, sinking them into the mud until they stood erect, their bright green tips pushing through the surface. The water was teaming with long, serpentine worms, snaking through our ankles and hands like ribbons of white.

I asked Nirina and Colette about them, as we planted the new rice shoots. "They're everywhere, now," Nirina said, "but they aren't so bad in the *tavy* fields. They like the water."

"We are used to them," Colette laughed, scooping up a handful of muddy water and watching the worms wash over her hands. She laughed at the look of disgust that came over my face.

"What do you mean, Nirina," I asked, "that they are everywhere *now*? Has it changed?"

"Oh, we've always had worms," she said, making a dismissive sound with her lips, "but now that we are working more in the rice fields, we have more than we had *taloha*." Again, that vague but common word for the indefinable past.

"You will get used to them, too," Colette laughed, "and your face will stop looking like that!"

Later that evening I asked Lalao, the woman who cooked and catered to me, for her opinion. Her father, Rivo, controlled many of the rice fields.

"There aren't as many in the *tavy* fields," she agreed, "but if the workers wouldn't drink the water, they wouldn't get so many worms." Her own siblings suffered from coughing and scabies, and while I had no doubt that they, too, had worms, they weren't as obvious as among others.

I explained about other ways worms could be transmitted, from feet to hand to mouth. She agreed that that was probably one way they were spread.

"But there is not much we can do about it. We have to work in the rice fields. But the more money we make, the more *tavy* we can clear. So if we work more in the wet rice fields, we can farm more *tavy* rice, and then maybe there will be fewer worms with time."[14]

I reflected on this conversation as I sat with Toky, holding his bloated belly and looking to me with sad pleading eyes, from a face well suited to dramatic exaggeration. "I cannot get better," he said, "because I must sleep on the wet floor all alone. Now that I am sick, I can sleep with my mother, but when I begin to get better she will make me sleep alone again, so that she can sleep with iPaul." I knew he was hoping I'd offer my own dry home, but I feared losing my privacy altogether once he moved in. Selfishly, I offered my sympathies but not my help.

"You will get better," I promised, "and if you don't, we will get you to the hospital."

"But then I will not be able to go to *school*," Toky pleaded, desperately seeking an angle to get me to offer my home. "I will forget the English you have taught me, and you will forget the Malagasy I have been teaching you. You won't be able to finish your work."

I assured him that would never happen. I would be sure he didn't forget his English lessons, and he could continue coaching me.

---

14. Lalao's claim that increasing wealth through the expansion of irrigated rice fields supported Ferraro's (1994) claim that encouraging wet-rice expansion did not lead to a decline in swidden production as the RNPP hypothesized, but instead, became a means of increasing overall rice production. Lalao did not comment on how it was that more fields would be cleared with the prohibition of further burning, nor did I ask given that she was not a landowner herself. My own experience was that existing fields, and lands outside the boundary of the park, were absorbed by wealthier people who rented or bought the fields of their less wealthy neighbors. As such, increased wealth through the limited agricultural assistance offered by the project was more likely to foster the consolidation of landholdings among an elite few, increase wage work by former subsistence farmers, and increase production of *tavy* currently in fallow.

But he went home that night to sleep in the wet puddles that seeped through the cracks in the mud that were the walls of his home.

Toky did recover from his fever and cough, though his belly stayed bloated. Within a few weeks the cyclone beat his home senseless. Toky had just enough time to grab his school books and their only cooking pot while Colette snatched up iPaul and they burst out the door in the slamming rain, just as their home caved in. The next morning I dropped by with my camera, taking a picture of the pile of mud and sticks that was their home, Colette standing next to the pile, laughing sadly at yet another disaster in her life.

Toky began using my house to do his homework, but slept each night on a different dirt floor, rotating from neighbor to neighbor until my research concluded and his mother's work with me had finished. Then they returned to her natal home, her husband having divorced her when he found a younger wife. iPaul, like another of Colette's sons and so many of Toky's friends, would soon die.

These stories of chronic illness illustrate the way that discomfort and illness have been naturalized by many who, although not necessarily regarding themselves as "healthy," have surrendered to the futility of trying to combat so many health concerns. Plant medicines are used, but with the daily constancy of discomfort, finding and preparing medicines can be yet another chore in lives marked by interminable labor, if just to find water, cook a pot of rice, or earn enough to buy a bit of petrol for the comfort of a small flame burning in the night.

And while Nety's death did not arise from one of the more common chronic illnesses, her death was in all probability brought on by her lack of medicines to control her seizures. Nety was fully informed and aware of her epilepsy and the medicine that would control it. Contrary to views that the "Tanala" are hopelessly tied to superstitious beliefs regarding illness, the multiple explanations that were offered to account for her death never departed from the general acknowledgment that she had an illness that was treatable by Western medication which she could not afford.

Physician and anthropologist Paul Farmer has pointed to the ways in which "cultural" explanations are offered to account for health treatment strategies that obscure social inequalities preventing many people from accessing modern medicines. In discussing the case of a young Haitian woman suffering from malaria, and whose father had her removed from a health clinic because he believed her illness was caused by witchcraft, Farmer asks:

> Do these events speak to the power and integrity of Haitian cultural traditions? Or do they point instead to inequalities of access which mean that, in rural Haiti, understandings of acute

infectious disease even now evolve largely in the absence of effective interventions that are readily available to nonpoor Haitians? Is Marie's a story about rural "beliefs" or rather a story about poverty and its effects on health outcomes among people who share her circumstances? I've spoken about "selective blindness." When an observer witnesses the effects of structural injustice and sees little more than cultural difference, is this not a conflation of cultural difference and structural violence? (Farmer 1999:154).

Although of the wealthier lineage and closely tied to the village elites, if one can call farmers who themselves work so close to the bone "elites," as an unmarried mother Nety lacked the cash to spend on medicines, and did not have land of her own which she could employ toward income. As such, Nety's gender and youth countered any benefit her lineage bestowed upon her, and her ethnicity failed to account for the fact that her illness had not been treated. By all accounts, Nety had been taking Western medication to treat her epilepsy; with the birth of her child two years previously and another on the way, her medicines became a luxury she could no longer afford. Her family concurred that the plants and other substances available in or near the forest could not control her seizures as could the pills she had once obtained from the clinic in Ranomafana.

And Lanto, herself a virtually landless woman, for what was left of her land after selling it to Rivo was beyond her ability to farm once she became sick and her son went to work for Raymond, was also unable to purchase the medicines she believed would relieve her respiratory problems. From a lineage reputed to be descended from slaves, middle aged and unmarried, she was a social outcast, even if sister to the *mpanjaka*. Her lineage, gender, and marginality in the community contributed to minimal social support in maintaining her fields and restoring her health. Her poverty thus exacerbated, her lack of access to medicine, health care, and knowledge contributed to her chronic illness. That she lived as "Tanala" seemed to have little bearing on the treatment strategies she pursued; she herself showed little faith in the healing faculties of Rakoto who, like all the *ombiasa* of Ranotsara and nearby, was of the Zafinaraina lineage.

Conversely, Kala and Zanabelo both identified themselves as "Betsileo," but this ethnic affiliation did not correspond to a more Westernized concept of illness and healing, as the hierarchal ordering of ethnic categories would suggest. While Kala treated her children's scabies with local plants, she and her husband both remained unconcerned as the condition worsened and became infected. And the clinic nurse who treated them either accepted their interpretation of how the illness was caused and encouraged them not to clean the wounds, or they interpreted his advice to correspond to their beliefs. Moreover, while they did not seek out indigenous treatment for the condition, they did seek out the preventative powers of a local *ombiasa* (of Zanabelo's Zafinaraina lineage) to ward off *katry*, an indigenous diagnosis for fevers and seizures. These actions suggest that ethnic affiliation cannot be ascribed to indigenous explanations for health problems, nor to treatment strategies. The lineage of Kala and Zanabelo was more likely to explain their trust in the powers of their cousin, an *ombiasa*, than was their ethnic affiliation, but lineage alone could not explain their actions, as they handled each illness episode separately, seeking Western medicines when they were affordable and available (when I provided them or the funds to purchase the antibiotic injection), indigenous plants when the illness was deemed ordinary and treatable, and shamanic intervention when the illness was believed serious but unnatural, with cosmological origins.

Critical Medical Anthropology

From the perspective of critical medical anthropology, "health can be defined as *access to and control over the basic material and nonmaterial resources that sustain and promote life at a high level of satisfaction*" (Baer, Singer and Susser 1997:5, emphasis theirs). This concept of health is the concept that I embrace in this book in presenting access to medicines as a resource issue, while tempering the notion of a "high level of satisfaction" to the more rational objective of a reasonable level of comfort and satisfaction.

Baer, Singer and Susser (1997:5), focusing primarily on the United States and expressing less concern with cross-cultural health systems, suggest that

> While the ultimate character of health care systems is determined outside the health sector by dominant social groups, like heads of insurance companies and other large corporations, significant forms of struggle take place within this sector and help to shape its institutions. Consequently, an examination of contending forces in and out of the health arena that impinge on health and healing becomes an essential task in building a critical approach to health issues.

The studies presented by Baer, Singer and Susser (1997), however, take a top-down approach, in which political and economic forces press down upon people represented as having relatively little autonomy or power, thereby affecting health and health behavior. For example, in discussing the historical and social context of alcoholism, the authors provide detailed evidence and sound argument to show how alcoholism can be understood in relationship to social class relations, in which drinking serves to unite workers in solidarity, control workers for the service of production, provide meaning to workers whose lives have been rendered meaningless through the production process, and provide profits to capitalists through the commodification of alcohol. In this way, alcoholism can be understood as a health problem directly related to class relations.

Such an analysis is important toward an understanding of the social and historical roots of an international health problem. But alcoholism is also a health problem that permeates class boundaries. And although alcoholism is a health problem of the wealthiest and the poorest in society (and may well disproportionately affect those in the poorest strata), how it is experienced, and how it is understood, differs among classes. Moreover, alcoholism is a health problem that divides not only the classes, but also within social classes, it is experienced and understood differently, as gender, age, race, religion, and geographical location shape how alcohol is consumed, experienced, and understood. The competing interests and views within a social strata that shape the etiology and morbidity of alcoholism, shape other health problems as well.

As Baer, Singer and Susser's (1997) study of alcoholism reflects, much of the work in critical medical anthropology has focused on how health status, the health and illness experience, and health care, are shaped by the capitalist economy *imposing* its values and interests onto others, an approach that comes from dependency theories, in which post-colonial societies are alleged to have been made dependent upon the wealthy nations of the north (e.g. Frank 1969). Morgan (1984) argued that a reliance on dependency theory to explain health problems has prevailed in critical medical anthropology, citing Baer (1982), Morsy (1979), and Singer (1986) as providing some of the most important work in this area, but limiting their analyses to documenting the ways that capitalist expansion and penetration have adversely affected health and contributed to inequitable distribution of health resources.

Specifically, Morgan (1984) points out that dependency theorists, in explaining medical systems and health problems in developing nations, often define capitalism in terms of the market, in which commodification of products for profit is the defining attribute, rather than relationship to the means of production. Furthermore, she indicates that capitalism does not affect people in a society uniformly; how they are themselves related to the means of production, and the initiative they themselves take to resist or become integrated into the penetration of capitalist economic systems, is critical to an understanding of social processes regarding health and medicine.

While the dependency approach to critical medical anthropology has shown how local health status and healing systems are linked to the broader national and international political economy (e.g. Morsy 1996), the failure of critical medical anthropologists to consider local forms of resistance and agency has weakened their analysis. People not only resist pressure to change their beliefs and behaviors regarding health and health care, they also actively engage in forging and refashioning their own health beliefs and practices; in some ways, these actions are independent of outside influence, in other ways, outside influences are incorporated into indigenous systems in willful and creative ways.[15]

The tendency to view indigenous systems as passively responding to the pressures of capitalist society is also reflected in medical anthropology studies of indigenous societies that romanticize indigenous medical practices as innately practical, beneficial, and adaptive, while capitalist medicine, or biomedical systems, are portrayed as innately impractical, harmful, and maladaptive. For example, while detailing the many ways in which indigenous Mayan childbirth practices provide a culturally-appropriate and woman-centered birthing experience, Jordan (1993) indicts Western biomedicine for creating a childbirth experience that ignores the needs and concerns of women, relies almost exclusively on biomedical technology that is presented as more harmful than helpful, and subordinates the knowledge of the indigenous practitioner, or the woman giving birth, to the authoritative knowledge of the Western practitioner. Her critiques are important ones and her cross-cultural analysis (in which she compares birthing systems in four different cultures) is both rare and enlightening, but by drawing such broad conclusions about biomedicine, one disregards the ways in which biomedicine can improve infant and maternal mortality and health. As Rhodes (1996) has shown, biomedicine is itself a cultural system, and as such, it merits respect and consideration.

In more recent work, anthropologists drawing on political economy of health approaches, or critical medical anthropology, have recognized that as much as biomedicine is a hegemonic cultural system, it is also in many ways, an efficacious one. For example, Millen, Irwin and Kim (2000) suggest that globalization has intensified social inequality, and that health indicators provide the most telling evidence for the uneven effects which economic and political changes have had on the world's population. They indicate that as technology and knowledge have increased significantly in the field of health, access to this technology and knowledge remains limited to certain groups of people. For those who lack such access, health

---

15. Farmer (1999), however, points out that much of social science and public health discourse has over-emphasized personal and collective "agency" to such an extent that the political and economic structures shaping health and disease are obscured.

care is not only limited, but health status remains low. For example, malnutrition affects 11.2 million people in the United States, and 828 million in post-colonial societies. Recognizing that proper nutrition helps to prevent disease, the authors point out that half of the 31,000 children under five who die each day, half die from hunger-related causes. In Africa, these rates have more than doubled since the mid 1980's, a period which coincides with the introduction of economic liberalization and structural adjustment policies.

Millen, Irwin and Kim (2000) conclude that indicators of economic growth must include health indicators, and that these indicators must consider multiple criteria, such as access to safe drinking water and sanitation, safe and appropriate housing, and disease prevention. Utilizing aggregate statistics to portray overall health status of a population may obscure the ways in which gains in some areas are offset by declines in others.

Contrary to presenting biomedicine as a hegemonic medical system that undermines indigenous medical systems, Kim, Millen, Irwin and Gershman (2000) present, in their edited volume, a number of case studies drawing on a political economy of health perspective which contend that biomedicine saves lives, and that political and economic development which intensifies the separation of the rich from the poor and makes access to this biomedicine the privilege of the minority, is untenable and immoral, a point that Farmer (1999) eloquently makes in his discussion of how treatable infectious diseases such as tuberculosis continue to kill millions of poor people every year.

While Morsy (1996:27) suggests that connecting "poor health to the inaccessibility of "Western" medicine obscures [the connections between the local, national and international levels]," I share with Kim, et al. (2000) the conviction that inaccessibility to Western medicines does contribute to poor health, and that lack of such medicines alone does not explain poor health. Other significant processes contribute to poor health, including economic changes imposed by national and international governments and institutions, as well as local power relations, and the cultural context in which the body and the environment are experienced and made meaningful.

In the following chapter, I continue this discussion of experience and meaning by illustrating how the medical belief systems of the people of Ranotsara are anything but homogenous. Competing, contradictory, and confusing explanatory models of illness and treatments to restore health are alive and well among these People of the Forest.

Chapter 8

Life and Death in Ranotsara

This chapter focuses on the multiple explanatory models and treatment strategies employed in the community of Ranotsara, suggesting that the concept of an indigenous medical system is problematic. Moreover, the variety of beliefs and practices that comprise the local response to illness is not at all related to one's ethnicity; rather, lineage, age, gender, and class are far more salient variables. Beliefs and practices related to health and healing are further conditioned by the access one has to health resources. The relationship one has to productive farming land, labor, and cash income, is the most important factor shaping one's health; this economic role further shapes how the relationship between the forest environment and health is perceived and experienced. Nonetheless, despite differences among community members in terms of health and material comfort, even the most land-rich of residents are impoverished by Western standards and this impoverishment, combined with limited access to Western health resources, have contributed to illness and death for all.

Treating, and Not Treating, Illness

Baoroa sits on a plank of wood that is her bed on the second floor of her family's home. The walls and thatched ceiling are lacquered from smoke; a small fire burns in the corner of the room over which a pot of rice is cooking. In her eighties and widowed for several years, Baoroa's days are spent cooking, caring for her grandchildren and greatgrandchildren, and resting—shortness of breath and severe arthritis limit her activities outside the home. She says it has been over a year since she has been to the river to bathe.

Baoroa's husband was a well-respected *ombiasa*, although she won't admit this to the *vazaha*. What she will say is that her husband's ancestors were among the *andriana* founders of the village, and as such, her social status is very high, a status she holds with pride as the eldest matriarch of the family. At her feet sits the wife of her grandson; the young woman, Jeanine, has brought her eighteen-month-old son from a distant village to consult her mother-in-law regarding the health of her boy.

The boy appears to be no older than six or seven months. His thin legs are folded like little chicken wings on which he sits, his arms are like tiny twigs. Next to him, his cousin iPaul, who was born just two weeks before him, rests on his mother's lap. Colette, iPaul's mother, rarely without a side-splitting laugh bursting from her mouth, is now very grave. She puts her fingers around iPaul's leg, to show how fat her boy is. Jeanine, in good humor, pinches the sagging skin from her own son's thighs to show off the comparison.

"He is too *kamo* (lazy) to walk," she says, as if this explains his skinny legs. His head rolls limply back to stare at the shiny black ceiling. "He should be more like iPaul."

"*Tsy ampy vitamine!*" Baoroa explodes in disgust ("Not enough vitamins!") and Colette echoes the sentiment, "*Tsy ampy*," shaking her head. Jeanine merely smiles, and continues her task.

She is mixing an ochre-colored paste of crushed roots from the wild ginger plant (*tamo-tamo*), with water, and dabbing it on her child. Baoroa instructs her in the proper method. First, the paste is rubbed on the child's fontanel; next, it is rubbed in bands around the neck, arms, and thighs, "where he is *manify-be* [very thin]," Colette explains. "She did not do this when the child was born, and so *biby* [ghosts] have entered the baby. "That is why he is so sick."

Later in the day there was much discussion among the women regarding the baby's illness. I wondered why it was that if the family believed the baby did not have enough vitamins, rather than give him food they painted his body with crushed roots.

"Baoroa said that he did not have enough vitamins. Do you believe that is why he is sick?" I asked a small group of women who had come to my house for tea by the fire.

"Yes, *tsy ampy vitamine*," Lalao said with sadness, as Nirina shook her head sadly in agreement, "*tsy ampy....*" she concurred.

"Why don't they feed him? Because they don't have enough money?"

"No, they are very rich," Colette responded in envy, "Did you see her nice clothes, that warm sweater she wears? She has many fine clothes, like you. They have much land, and many crops, and they eat *laoka* [sauce, usually of greens or beans, that is served on rice] every day. They are not too poor."

"Then why don't they feed him?" I asked, bewildered.

"I don't know the reason," Lalao answered, "She also has a daughter, and she is very fat."

"Maybe she thinks girls are better than boys." I suggested.

"No!" Nirina protested, shaking her head vigorously, "Tanala love *all* babies."

"Yes," Lalao agreed, "there is no difference. But when he was small, he was very sick. Maybe she thinks that there is no reason to feed him because he will die. After he was sick, he became weaker and weaker, and maybe she thought he would die."

"Does this happen often?" I wondered, "people don't feed their babies if they think they will die?"

"No, not often. But maybe that is the reason," explained Lalao, "I don't know why she does not feed him. She is not wise [*tsy mahay izy*].

"If she would not feed him, why didn't the family do or say something?"

"Because that is not our affair [*tsy ny raharahan' izahay*]," answered Colette, Jeanine's sister-in-law, "It is the business of the mother and father to feed their children."

"But it was different in the past," Nirina added, "In the past, if a child was hungry, the family would give him food, but now, life is hard, there is not enough money and not enough food. People eat in their homes and do not share much food because there is not much to share."

"No, there is not enough," Colette agreed.

I often heard about the better life *taloha*, in the past, and though I asked, it was never clear how far in the past it was when things were better nor if life really was better in the past, or if memories had made it so.

"But if he is sick because he doesn't have enough vitamins," I asked, "why are they giving him the *tamo tamo*?"

"Maybe there is another reason he is sick," Lalao suggested, "Maybe Rakoto will cure him. He is knowledgeable [*mahay*] about the illnesses of the spirits [*aretina biby*]. That is why they took him to see Rakoto."

Rakoto had accepted the mantle of *ombiasa* with the passing of his father, a few years before. Well versed in ceremonial, learned from his father, his own knowledge of local illness categories and the plants used for treating them was either very limited, or it was his willingness to share his knowledge with me that was limited.

But Rakoto could not cure the baby, he later confessed to me, because the parents had waited too long before applying the *tamo-tamo*. By waiting so long, he explained, the soft-spot on the top of his head had grown so big it reached the child's forehead. So Rakoto sent the child to Letsara, a man who lived in a village in the hills above Ranotsara, and was known for his expertise with *ody loha* [head medicine, or the medicine used to seal the soft spot; noted for being different for each family].

Letsara gave the baby a tea, and made an inhalation for the child, but it was never revealed to me which plants were used. He also made a paste from *fandrinkabodisa*, a thorny vine found in the secondary growth outside the forest, and added it to the *tamo-tamo*, again painting bands on the wrists, knees, and ankles, and covering the soft-spot.

"Rakoto told them to use the *tamo tamo*," Lalao continued. "Maybe the baby will be able to walk if they use the *tamo tamo*."

"But he cannot walk because he needs food," I said, having difficulty accepting painting the baby with roots as an effective treatment for starvation.

"He cannot walk because his legs are too thin," Colette patiently explained to me. "Our babies were born at the same time, but she did not eat much even when she was pregnant. Then her baby became sick and he didn't eat much. iPaul eats all the time!" she laughed as we watched him struggle with a banana, "and so he has fat legs and walks all the time. But her baby is too weak to walk, he is not strong at all. He is too weak to eat. If he has *vary* [rice], he spits it out. He cannot even eat *vary*. Maybe the spirits have made him sick because she did not follow the *fomba* [custom] of putting the *tamo tamo* on his head when he was born. The spirits entered his body and have made him too sick to eat."

"She should give that baby *laoka!*" Nirina said in disgust, spitting out a wad of *paraky* [chewing tobacco] as she set down her empty tea cup and hobbled off to find some booze.

By late afternoon the baby was unconscious. Baoroa and her eldest son, Rakotobe, agreed that the best thing to do was to send the baby to the hospital in Ranomafana for treatment, because he would surely die if he remained in the village. They would continue the *tamo tamo* treatment, however, because unless the *cause* of the baby's illness — his failure to eat — was not addressed, the *effects* of the illness would worsen.

Jeanine, accompanied by Rakoto and Rakotobe, who carried his grandson, reached the hospital by nightfall. The hospital physician diagnosed the child as suffering from malnutrition and dehydration. He was treated with antibiotics and vitamins, and told that there was no bed available for him to remain there. The family kept him with family in Ranomafana and while there he received many visitors. Jeanine obtained powdered milk (diluted with local water) and meals for the baby. She began feeding him watery rice (*vary lena*, rice served in its cooking water, and given to the sick), with *laoka*.

The baby regained consciousness and after three days in Ranomafana, Rakotobe carried him home, hiking the nine kilometers over the mountainous terrain. He reached the village by late afternoon, the limp baby wrapped in a blanket on the hot sunny day. Several villagers met him at the edge of the village to celebrate the return of the sick baby, following the family home to learn the news in Ranomafana and share the family's joy.

By the end of the night, the baby had died.

The Malagasy Medical System

Understanding the Malagasy medical system necessitates understanding that it does not exist. The very concept of a system — be it an eco-system, social system, or medical system—is a reified concept that exists solely in the mind of the observer. The observer selects, discards, arranges, categorizes, and ranks elements of the system in such a way as to discern patterns. In medicine, these elements can be observed as signs, symptoms, causes, processes, diagnoses, treatments and outcomes—how these elements are grouped and evaluated constitute the patterns of the medical system.

Medical anthropology has attempted to illuminate such patterns from their multiple perspectives, in order to better understand differing ways of conceptualizing health and illness that challenge our own perceptual patterns of health and illness. By focusing on alternative healing systems or indigenous knowledge systems, however, one is almost forced to think in terms of a shared concept of reality grounded in social structure and history. There is indisputable value in doing this, but nevertheless, individual experience, faith, character, intellect and knowledge penetrate the social system in such a way that no two individuals in a given society conceptualize the illness experience, nor their health needs, identically. Nirina, for example, viewed the illness of Jeanine's baby in terms of nutrition, while Rakoto viewed it in terms of social discord, specifically, the violation of the *fomba* and the entry of malevolent spirits.

Were these differing views related to the social roles of Nirina, an elderly female who had lived in cities and had considerable exposure to colonial medicine, and Rakoto, a young male *ombiasa* trained in the use of forest medicines for treating illnesses caused by spirits? Perhaps. Nonetheless, Baoroa, at least as old as Nirina, viewed the illness in much the same way as did Rakoto, that is, in terms of social discord, even though Baoroa acknowledged the baby needed "vitamins." Baoroa's deceased husband, and now her grandson, were well respected *ombiasa*. Nirina, conversely, while she herself was regarded as knowledgeable regarding plant medicines for children, and covertly visited *ombiasa*, considered herself a devout Catholic. At least publicly, she would promote the use of Western medicines and vitamins for the child. That there is a multiplicity of views and explanations for illness and healing in Ranotsara, is as true in the forests of Madagascar as it is in any town or city of the United States. But I found no evidence co-relating differences in these views to one's ethnic identity. Just as concepts of health and healing in the United States are understood in terms of education, family income, and social power, so too did I find these same factors having more to bear on explanatory models in Ranotsara than did ethnic identity. For example, Baoroa and Rakoto were among the few in the village who identified themselves as "Betsileo," and tied this identity to their social status as *"andriana-be"* [very royal], a status they claimed due to their descent from the Zafinaraina line that was not tainted by the marriage to *andevo*. Nirina, conversely, reported that she had

once been "Betsileo," but became "Tanala." It is not clear if her change in
ethnic status was associated with her marriage to Faly, a Zafindraraoto, or
her many years of living the "Tanala" life of the forest. What was clear
was that she continued to identify her ancestry as "Betsileo," but regarded
her age and experience as a rural farmer and woman to be the defining
characteristics by which both her "Tanala" ethnicity and her world views
were formed. Nonetheless, ethnic identity, as I've indicated previously, is
fluid. It was not at all uncommon to find a person identifying themselves
with a particular ethnic group one moment, and with another the next.

My point is not that there is no cultural foundation to perceptions of
health and healing in Ranotsara, but that this cultural foundation is not an
"ethnic" one. While I use the term "Tanala" to refer to the people of whom
I write, and in this way, may speak of a "Tanala medical system" or "Tanala
culture," I am using the term in the same way that those who live in Ranotsara use it—to refer to the "people of the forest," those who live and
work and die among the forested hills of southeastern Madagascar. A fundamental feature of the culture arising from their shared histories and
lifestyles, is social differentiation based on gender, age, and lineage. The belief that these social differences are important ones, that one's gender, age,
or lineage defines not just who one is, but what rights one has to resources
and social networks, is a cultural belief, and contributes to distinctive cultural practices, including beliefs and practices about health and healing.

Crandon-Malamud (1991) persuasively argued that the quest for health
resources leads people to negotiate their identities by way of shifting ethnic, religious and cultural features in such a way that they position themselves to better access health care and medicines. In her view, by distinguishing "medical systems" as having fixed boundaries such as
"indigenous," "cosmopolitan," "Western" or "folk," one may lose sight
of the ways that people exchange knowledge, draw from multiple health
"systems," and continually recast their social identities to increase the
treatment options available to them.

By glossing particular beliefs or practices as "cultural," moreover, without regard to the multiplicity of beliefs and practices associated with the
culturally recognized categories of gender, age, or lineage, is misleading.
Culture cannot be separated from the power relations it fosters and re-
produces, nor from the broader political and economic processes affecting
these relations beyond the boundaries of the village. Conceptualizing the
cultural context of a medical system thus requires an understanding of the
historical, political, and economic processes that affect health, healing,
and social relations at the local level. In so doing, it becomes difficult to cling
tenaciously to the concept of the "medical system," a concept that Western science has distinguished from other cultural domains, such as the social, political, economic, and cosmological (see Morsy 1996).

By stepping outside the "medical system" to focus on individual variations, such as those expressed by Nirina and her close friend Baoroa, one is brought closer to understandings of power and the relationship between power and knowledge. Although having very different views regarding the illness of Jeanine's son, Nirina and Baoroa did not differ in any socially-relevant way except for the status brought them through their marriages. Nirina, having been born into the Zafinaraina lineage, a lineage locally represented as *andriana*, lost status with her marriage to Faly, while Baoroa, originally from Ranomafana, gained status through her marriage into the Zafinaraina. Ironically, it was the marriage of a Zafinaraina (Ramistiry) to a Zafindraraoto (iKalahafa) in the previous generation which elevated the status of Baoroa's husband, because his descent from Ramistiry's brother, Ndrianomy (who married a woman alleged to be *andriana*), rendered him "more pure" than his cousins. This single accident of heritage became a defining attribute to one's identity in Ranotsara, as the family of Baoroa visibly separated itself from the more materially-advantaged family of Rivo (grandson of Ramitsiry), even maintaining a separate *tranobe* so that burial of their dead would remain undefiled by either the Zafindraraoto or those who married them.

As their material status diminished in comparison to their cousins (Rivo, Philippe and Pascal), however, it became even more important for the family of Baoroa to adhere to the social supremacy of ancestry. The role of Rakoto as *ombiasa* therefore served as a direct conduit to this ancestral realm. It was not surprising then, that in explaining the malnutrition of their kin, they would focus on this violation of tradition, while Nirina herself took the more pragmatic approach and suggested the child needed food.[1] The ease with which Nirina expressed this view might also be related to the fact that because she was outside the immediate family, she was not as concerned with the stigma of shame such a statement might provoke. As Howard and Millard (1997) have suggested in their analysis of malnutrition on Mt. Kilimanjaro, for one's child to be malnourished is a great source of shame for the Chagga. At the time of my research I had not considered the concept of shame and its cultural context among the Malagasy; nonetheless, in retrospect there might well have been a sense of shame influencing the parents' delay in seeking treatment for their son, and might help explain why the child's family reflected on social offenses. Although a violation of social custom might also carry a stigma, to violate a *fady*

---

1. Maurice Bloch (personal communication 2001) has questioned my analysis of this case, suggesting that other health problems probably contributed to the child's death. His judgment is persuasive and plausible; nonetheless, lacking access to medical records of the village and of this child, I was only able to draw on conjectures of village residents for my analysis.

requires a certain degree of agency, and therefore does not have the association with victimization and powerlessness that comes with malnutrition.

Thirty years ago, Glick (1967) raised the issue of power in terms of medical anthropology and medical systems, in his discussion of ideas regarding sources of disease-causing power. "One must learn where people believe power to reside or inhere; and one must learn how they endeavor to put it to their own uses" (Glick 1967:34). Ancestry has become this locus of power in Ranotsara, and reflects some similarities to Glick's own findings.

Glick's study of a medical system in the New Guinea highlands used the concept of power to understand how health and illness were patterned and experienced among the Gimi. By focusing on medicines as having social power, Glick showed that the local pharmacopeia extended beyond the "efficacious" substances a Westerner might regard as significant. He found that illness, as a social process evoking a response within the medical system, determines health needs. As such, medicinal "needs" extend well beyond those remedies judged as valuable by Western researchers, and the therapeutic substances thus sought by the Gimi, as by others, are possessed of a power to heal, whether that power be measurable in the laboratory or not. For Baoroa, the yellow-ochre powder of the *tamo-tamo* root possessed a social power that Nirina's *laoka* [sauce] did not.

As Jeanine's son suffered from malnutrition (undoubtedly complicated by other, undiagnosed, health problems) and the family sought—in differing ways—strategies for treating his illness, another member of the community fell sick. Solo was a young man, in his early twenties, recently married and the father of a young boy. As the eldest grandson of Kotomahay, in line for the position of *mpanjaka* of the Zafindraroato lineage, Solo's social status was among the highest of his age-mates; his economic status, however, was among the lowest. He and his wife, Celine, and their son, Jean Elie, lived in a small one-room house, about three meters by three meters. The house was in poor repair and offered minimal protection against the heavy rains. They had very little land, which did not produce enough food for the family. Indeed, their crops and income were so minimal that they often went without meals altogether. Jean Elie, about four months of age, was severely malnourished, looking barely more than four weeks old. His yellowed skin was covered with scabies lesions he'd had since birth, and his scalp was raw from untreated cradle cap which had turned to open sores and become severely infected.

Seventeen year old Celine had one year of schooling, and could neither read nor write. She was regarded among the other women in the community as very nice but extremely naive, not even understanding, some women giggled, how it was that she had become pregnant when she began sleeping with Solo.

In mid-July, Solo fell ill late in the day. After working for wages in the fields of the Zafinaraina, he began to feel cold and his head ached. By early evening, his chest was hurting, and by the following morning, his stomach hurt, he had diarrhea, and his legs were sore. Throughout the morning his whole body hurt, and he described the pain as moving all over his body. By noon, however, his headache had cleared and the pain had settled in his stomach and the bones and joints of his legs.

The description Solo gave of his illness, as having begun in his head and progressed to his chest, then his stomach, then legs, led his family to conclude that this was an unusual illness marked by a unique progression from his head downward. This was clearly not an illness of God, but instead, suggestive of either *mpamosavy* (witchcraft) or punishment of the ancestors. Therefore, it was necessary to consult an *ombiasa*.

Naina was called in to diagnose Solo's illness the first night he fell ill. He arrived at about eight in the evening, after dark. He said he found Solo unconscious, and the family told him that Solo had been trembling. Not knowing the illness, he consulted the *sikidy*. The *sikidy* is a divination system introduced by Arab traders in the fifteenth century. Linton (1933:203) suggests that the term *sikidy*, when used by the Tanala Ikongo, refers to all types of divination, including divination by water, sand or mirror, as well as by seeds. My own experience, however, was that in the region of Ranotsara, the term referred solely to divination by seeds, which Linton suggests is how the Tanala Menabe use the term. (When asked about the difference, the residents of Ranotsara indicated to me that they were unfamiliar with the ethnic distinctions of Tanala Ikongo and Tanala Menabe.)

According to the *sikidy*, Naina explained, Solo's illness was very grave and had been sent by the ancestors to punish him for the way he had been treating his grandfather, Kotomahay. Naina asked Kotomahay if Solo had upset him, and Kotomahay replied that he and Solo had been fighting because Solo was not behaving like a grandson and showing him proper respect. Naina explained that in order to restore Solo's health, his grandparents, Kotomahay and Soary, had to show forgiveness by blessing Solo with water in which the leaves and stems of the *maniny* tree (found in the forest), and raw white rice, were added. In so doing, he explained, the ancesters would be satisfied that order was restored.

While the *ombiasa* and the family were unanimous in believing the illness to be caused by the ancestors, they at the same time believed that the cold, rainy weather caused the symptoms of the illness. In effect, Kotomahay explained, the ancesters were upset with Solo, and therefore, by attacking his strength, or immunity, caused him to be susceptible to an illness brought by the weather. Consequently, Naina also prescribed a tea made from the leaves and roots of *ahibalala*. As discussed in the previous chapter, *ahibalala* is a plant that grows in the *tavy* fields and is known by virtually everyone in the village as an all-purpose cold and flu remedy. Family members explained that it was very effective for *tazo*, or fever, and works in the same way that Niviquine works in treating fevers. Moreover, it was said to be effective for stomach disorders, and so he thought that it would help Solo's fever and stomach upset.

Consequently, Naina's treatment was aimed at not only restoring social order (the cause of the illness), but at healing the symptoms of the illness as well. My visit, however, altered the treatment strategy of the family. The moment I began asking questions regarding the medicines Solo had taken, I was asked for aspirin. I explained that although I had aspirin, I did not know if it would be a good medicine for Solo's illness, because it would upset his stomach. Kotomahay, a village elder whose knowledge of plant medicines was well respected in the community, asked if I could give his grandson something else, if aspirin were not effective. Although I reminded the villagers, almost daily, that I was not a *doctera*, and they did understand the limits to my knowledge, there was no escaping the fact that I had medicines. I indicated that I had Nautamine, which was effective for treating upset stomachs, though it would not really treat his illness. No matter, Kotomahay thought Solo should give it a try. As such, I did give Solo some Nautamine, and within moments of swallowing the bitter pill, he rose from his sickbed and announced that he was much better.

But Solo was far from better, and as the day progressed, his family determined that he needed to recover from the illness in order to fully regain his strength. He spent the following week huddled in a dark corner of his grandfather's home, receiving visitors. His grandmother cooked for him, though he ate very little. Chickens were killed and boiled, and Solo was served the meat and broth for his strength. But his illness, rather than diminishing, grew stronger, and soon he was coughing. Meanwhile, his grandfather, Kotomahay, also took sick with a headache, and stripping off his clothes and wrapping himself in a burial shroud, he, too, huddled in a corner of his home, moaning audibly as he received visitors. While Kotomahay indicated that he had the same symptoms as Solo, he told me that he did not think the illnesses were related, but that he was having a heart attack.

Village gossip, however, suggested that Kotomahay did indeed think his illness was related to his grandson's sickness. Shortly before Solo fell ill, there had been a Saturday night drinking bout among some young men in the nearby market town of Masomanga. After many glasses of *toaka gasy*, a healthy young man fell into a coma and died shortly after. His death, like all deaths from *toaka* ingestion, was attributed to *mosavy*, or witchcraft. Legend has it that several years back someone from Ranotsara had died after drinking the *toaka* brought by a visitor from Masomanga.

That visitor was thereby marked as a *mpamosavy* [witch], as was the woman who headed the household he was visiting in Ranotsara. Death from *toaka*, something people drank daily, was not regarded as normal. Withcraft was obvious.

As such, the death from *toaka gasy*, in a healthy young man no less, was judged by many people to be the work of a witch, and that witch was undoubtedly the woman in Ranotsara who had hosted the stay of the visitor who had poisoned the *toaka gasy* he brought to Ranotsara several years back. In revenge for the recent death in Masomanga, some villagers speculated, a *mpamosavy* had probably been called upon to curse someone in Ranotsara. Solo's illness, therefore, marked him, and his family, as somehow linked to this *mosavy* business (while no one would name the witch, I was told that she was already grown and her husband had left her; that she was said to be of the *andevo* [slave] caste was also significant.)

Consequently, there were two simultaneous explanations for Solo, and then his grandfather, falling ill — one was that the ancestors were displeased with the way that Solo treated his grandparents and had cursed him with an illness — Kotomahay's response to Solo was regarded by the ancestors as equally disgraceful, and so he too was struck down. The other interpretation was that Solo and Kotomahay had been struck ill to avenge the *mosavy* death of the young man in Masomanga.

Kotomahay recovered, while Solo, either for his recovery or protection, it was never really clear to me, was sent to distant relatives where he could have "new air." Within a few months, however, Solo's son died from malnutrition, never having been served the chicken that was sacrificed for his father. Celine told me she did not have enough milk for the baby, and the food for the family was so scarce they could not give any to the baby, who was too weak to chew rice. "*Ahibalala*," she told me, "is the only medicine I know."

My initial reaction to these illness episodes was to wonder why it was that Solo's illness — which from my perspective appeared to be a common flu — received so much attention, while his son's apparent malnutrition remained neglected. The community did not hesitate to rally for Solo, yet did nothing to intervene with his son's health, just as no one would intervene to care for Jeanine's seemingly malnurished son — except to paint rings around his twig-like limbs. How could the community allow children to apparently starve while adults with upset stomachs were nursed day and night?

The answers to these questions came bit by bit over the next few months, as Solo slowly recovered, and his son continued to waste away. While I focused on what I perceived to be ignorance — a failure of people to recognize the severity of malnutrition as compared to vague aches and pains, the people of the community focused on issues of power. And much of that power centered on one's relationship to the forest, that is, how one was, or was not, empowered to control the land and resources of the forest that surrounded them.

Although Solo's grandfather was a well-respected community elder in line for the position of *mpanjaka* of the Zafindraraoto lineage, the inflation of recent years contributed to the economic disempowerment of Solo's family such that Kotomahay was frequently forced to labor in the fields of Rivo, Philippe, or Pascal for wages of 1,500 fmg a day (approximately 35 cents at the time of my fieldwork). Nonetheless, Kotomahay regarded himself as better off economically than when he was younger, because his children were grown and he was no longer responsible for their care, despite the fact that he continued to feed several of his children and grandchildren. And although he had good irrigated rice fields, as each son married, he gave them their own land, thereby reducing his own land holdings.

Unable to expand his *tavy* fields into the newly-created national park, Kotomahay's access to land and forest resources did not expand as his children matured and took possession of their lands. Compounded with the escalating cost of living, Kotomahay's wages became necessary for family survival. Similarly, each of his sons, and his remaining daughters, was forced into wage labor for the Zafinaraina as well. The result of Kotomahay and his grown children working for wages while simultaneously working their irrigated and swidden rice fields, was that they had less labor available to assist in their own fields and their harvests subsequently declined. Declining harvests led to the need to borrow rice from the Zafinaraina, which were repaid in double the following years. As such, much of their own lands were devoted to growing rice for the Zafinaraina.

Therefore, by the time Solo married and took possession of his rice fields, there were no other family members available to help him and Celine work the lands, while Solo also found himself assisting in clearing the lands and harvesting the crops of the Zafinaraina lineage, in order to have cash income. The result was that Solo had access to land, but lacking access to labor and his own labor sold for wages, he was unable to maximize the production of his land. In short, he was extremely poor, and did not have enough food to feed himself, his wife, and his son.

Had community members intervened by calling attention to Jean Elie's poor health and emaciation, they would have had to confront the fact that Solo was unable to feed him because he and his family were economically disempowered, and their labor power was therefore devoted to wage work, rather than working their own lands. As such, their relationship to the land had changed with the changing social and economic structure of the village.

As for ignoring the fundamental reasons they were impoverished and simply giving food to the boy, community members expressed the fear that to give food to others during periods of scarcity would cause them to become malnourished themselves. Kotomahay himself told me that this was a recent phenomena; during his parents' time, food and resources were shared and those who lacked were provided for by those who had more. But why, then, didn't Kotomahay or his sons give food to the boy? I do not really know; Kotomahay was a kind and generous man. Perhaps he and his family had internalized the fear of going without.

Kotomahay expressed his frustrations at not having the power to care for his family, despite his role as village elder and future *mpanjaka*. His own sense of disempowerment was reflected in his conflict with Solo—feeling that his grandson did not respect his authority, he promoted the view that the ancestors had weakened Solo as punishment, just as he later accepted the view that Solo's illness may have been caused by the ever-powerful *mpamosavy* of Masomanga. This latter view explained why he, too, became sick and thereby "disempowered" even more. Feeling weakened economically, socially, and cosmically, it is not that difficult to accept that Kotomahay and others in his family may have felt that they lacked the power to help Jean Elie, whose wasting was a reflection of the family's loss of power.[2]

Conversely, Jeanine's son had apparently starved to death, despite his family's economic power. And while his wasting and death prompted much speculation and difference of opinion, it did not prompt much intervention. Is it that children are regarded as unimportant? Quite the contrary, a child's death, while commonplace, is regarded as a terrible tragedy. But to intervene with how a parent cares for their child is to subvert their most fundamental power, that is, the power to care for one's family, while contesting an even greater power—the power of the ancestors to intervene. As economic power diminished for nearly everyone, families came to rely more and more on the power of the ancestors to take care of social problems, because most people viewed themselves as socially disempowered with the changing economy.

Another factor contributing to the failure of the community to act, was that Jeanine's husband was regarded as *andriana*; those who were allegedly *andevo* could not intervene, while malnutrition was not regarded as an illness of the *andriana*. It had to be something else. Respecting the power of the spiritual world, it was understandable that the spirits would enter the boy's body and make him sick. And if Lalao was correct in her view that after the boy had become sick, his mother felt that there was nothing she could do to help him to survive, her own sense of disempowerment may have contributed to his demise.

---

2. I offer these explanations as my own, possibly mistaken, interpretations and they may or may not accord with those of the people to whom I imply them.

Despite the conflicting views as to where power resided in respect to the boy's health and sickness, whether it be in *tamo tamo*, the parents, the spirits, or the hospital, the consensus was that for others to feed Jeanine's son, when she and her husband could afford to feed him, would take limited food away from one's own family. Howard and Millard (1997:8) noted the same pattern of neglect in their study of the malnutrition in East Africa, arguing that "In the period of food crisis, many sought to protect the members of their own households by denying assistance to poorer kin who had little to offer in return in the cash economy." In Ranotsara, those without land or cash resources could only offer their labor in exchange for assistance.

At the same time that kin turned their back on the plight of Jeanine's child, to suggest to Jeanine that she feed him would be rude. To call on the ancestors for intervention, however, would enable the child to receive care. Moreover, in so doing, the power of biomedicine and the power of forest medicines were invoked as his care gained the attention of both *ombiasa* and the hospital physician.

In this case, the family had access to indigenous medicines, particularly through the family connection to Rakoto and Baoroa. Yet in the early stages of the boy's life and sickness, they rejected it. Family members allege that the mother — an outsider from a different village — lacked access to knowledge, that she, as the primary caretaker of the child, was ignorant. Her ignorance, it was said, explained her failure to eat well during pregnancy, to follow the *fomba* of protecting the fontanel with *tamo tamo*, and to feed the baby adequately.

Thus, the undernourishment and deaths of two babies, one from the Zafindraraoto lineage, the other from the Zafinaraina lineage, were viewed and interpreted differently by the community. Jean Elie's death was regarded as related to poverty, and he wasted away slowly, with no intervention at all. The death of Jeanine's son, of the Zafinaraina lineage, was regarded by many as a spiritual disorder, even by those, such as Baoroa, who felt the child did need "vitamins." As such, the healing power of forest medicines was sought, and when they failed, the healing power of the hospital was solicited. There appeared to be no effort to secure such power toward the healing of Jean Elie, perhaps because his family viewed itself, and was viewed by others, as socially and economically powerless.

To some, however, the illness and death in Kotomahay's family might be understood in terms of a "Tanala" ethnic identity, while the differing approach to the sickness and death of Jeanine's baby might be conceptualized in terms of her family's declared "Betsileo" ancestry. But to distinguish the differing illness strategies as reflecting differing ethnic views of medicine, would be misleading because it would obscure the ways in which poverty and local kinship ties mediate the illness experience in Ranotsara.

Different economic positions, accompanied by different familial ties, are more salient to how one explains and treats illness in Ranotsara, than are spurious ethnic differences.

Howard and Millard (1997) have pointed out that high rates of child malnutrition are not attributable to local people, nor to outside influences such as the global economy alone; rather, they suggest that it is the interaction of customary practices with these outside forces that shape local economics. In the case of Ranotsara, the customary practices that interacted with the global economy were those related to a division of labor based on descent, in which those members of the Zafinaraina lineage were better positioned to call on their wealthier kin for assistance, while those of the Zafindraraoto lineage faced a continuing decline in economic security, further compounded by the Park's enclosure of lands they regarded as their rightful heritage. Moreover, Howard and Millard (1996:xv) note that

> The shift to commodity food production has been accompanied by weakening reciprocity between the poor and their community leaders, by an increasing gap between rich and poor, and by the growing poverty of many households faced with shortages of farmland and landlessness.

But landlessness alone, or even in association with close kinship ties to the ruling lineage, does not explain all poverty in Ranotsara, just as poverty alone does not explain all sickness. Gender and access to labor further exacerbate poverty, as the following story reveals, while lack of access to medicines, health care, and health knowledge, combine with the tropical environment to exacerbate chronic illness.

Explanatory Models for A Culture-Bound Diagnosis

As discussed previously, Rivo and his brother Koto launched the land consolidation that currently characterizes Ranotsara. But as their business savvy and good fortune were blessing them with the riches of abundant crops and cattle and a bit of cash, the fortunes of their elder brother, Lita, were not as prosperous. As the eldest brother, Lita had received the largest and finest rice fields from their father, but in middle age, his eyesight began to fail. By the time of my arrival, as Rivo and Koto had already established their wealth, Lita's eyesight was virtually gone. He could no longer tend his fields, and the only contribution he could make to the household was to chop the wood each day, a task he carried out by touch, rather than by sight.

Having lost the ability to manage his fields or contribute to the household economy, the responsibility fell to his wife, Soa.

When Soa married Lita, she was in her late twenties, with two children from a previous marriage, and another child already buried. She left her first husband, she explained, because he was lazy, and did not take care of his children. In contrast, Lita publicly adopted Soa's remaining child, Ketaka. Soa and Lita then had four more children, three boys and one girl, as Lita gradually went blind.

My arrival in Ranotsara was delayed by three days, however, when one of their boys died of apparent respiratory failure, and a funeral was held. Within a few months, another son was gone, again of apparent respiratory failure. Soa, having given birth to six children, was left with only three surviving children, Ketaka, Lala, and Chantelle. At the age of thirty-one, her husband blind and unable to work, Soa had little time to mourn her children because it was up to her and her children to farm her land.

Having no adult relatives of her own to call on to help her farm, and Lala and Chantelle too young to do much, Soa and Lita turned to Lita's brother, Rivo, and offered to lease their irrigated rice fields to him for a period of three years in exchange for 50,000 fmg (about $12.50). They knew that this sum was significantly less than the value of the land, which Lala speculated would yield crops valued at up to 250,000 fmg a year, but with no one they could call on to help with the labor, no cash with which to pay hired laborers, and no other bidders for land in the community, the couple's options were limited. With the 50,000 fmg they received, Soa was able to buy clothing and school supplies for the children, and some food, but she did not have enough to set aside.

She continued to work their *tavy* fields alone, but when she was in need of cash, she left her own fields to work for wages for Rivo. Ketaka and Chantelle also helped Rivo; as their father's brother, they were expected to treat him with the same respect as they would show to their father. In their case, this meant working in his fields regularly, without pay, and every afternoon, after school let out, going to Rivo's rice fields to watch for birds, which they scared away with slingshots and stones. Although the girls received no pay, in consideration of their labor Rivo provided them with regular meals. The labor of the girls also served as a sort of social insurance, in case Soa came to him in the future in need. Thus, while relinquishing her fields for such low pay could be perceived as victimization, to Soa renting out the fields, in conjunction with "loaning" out the labor of her children, increased her options and her potential leverage with her brother-in-law.

But Soa's needs grew greater as her work wore away at her body and her poverty dragged her down. She was the only person in the village who appeared depressed. She rarely smiled, and did not pretend to be happy, unless she was drunk. She often drank *toaka gasy*, as did many women, and though she could not afford to buy it for herself, others offered it to her, knowing it was for her a sort of medicine. Lita, however, did not approve of her drinking and they often fought over it when she returned home drunk.

"He is angry because I've been drinking *toaka gasy*," Soa giggled one evening, after a fight had sent her out of her house and over to mine, where several of the women had gathered. "Maybe he will divorce me, and then I'll have less work. He is sick again, you know, with *bay*."

Yes, I knew. Lita's chronic *bay* was providing me with rich data on forest medicines. *Bay* is generally a skin disorder; some use the term to refer only to swollen, pus-filled growths such as boils or carbuncles, others used the term to refer to any type of skin disorder not-otherwise recognized (such as scabies). Because the environment is anything but sterile, with feces prevalent throughout the village and surrounding areas, and clean water difficult to come by, the slightest break in the skin, such as from a mosquito bite, could become infected very quickly. In no time at all I was covered with my own *bay*, and my home became the local dispensary for antiseptic to cleanse everybody's budding *bay*.

Lita, however, did not come to me for help, sending Soa in his place to inquire after pills. One particularly crippling *bay* had taken root beneath his scapula. As it grew bigger and bigger, it became impossible for him to move his arm, and that meant that he could no longer chop wood. Rivo, however, did not come to Lita's aid, providing only periodic offerings of cooking wood. Lala and Ketaka took over that obligation, as well, collecting stray bits of wood on their way to and from the fields. Soa was also earning extra money by pounding rice for Rivo, for which she received 1,500 fmg a day.

"I want a divorce," Soa told me, still fuming about Lita's criticism of her drinking, "but I have nowhere to go, and I am too poor to leave the village. And if I divorce him, I cannot ask Rivo for help if I need it. Do you have anymore *toaka*? My glass is empty," and she chuckled some more. By five a.m. the next day she was back to work in Rivo's fields, earning cash to pay the *ombiasa* for Lita's treatment.

Naina stopped by to check on Lita every day, but the latter initially declined his assistance. Naina explained that Lita was suffering from *bay mainty*, "black *bay*," which was the most serious form. Soa would gather medicines in the *tavy* fields and prepare poultices for him, but by the time Lita agreed to Naina's treatment, his wound was very large and deep. Naina went to the forest for the branch of a tree, and stripping its bark, he plunged the end of the wooden pestle-shaped branch in the fire and held it firm to the wound. Repeating this treatment several times a day, along with Soa's home remedy, the wound eventually opened, and within a few days Lita was healed.

But Soa's problems continued to surmount. Within a few months, she was visibly pregnant, confessing that she was due at the same time as the rice, implying her fear that she would be unable to bring in her rice harvest. Adding to her daily work of farming her own fields, pounding rice for Rivo, periodically working his irrigated rice fields (which he had leased from her), she had begun working for me as well, to gain not only income, but my obligations toward her. Contrary to Malagasy "cultural" forms of discourse, in which participants seek to put the other at ease by remaining cheerful and by approaching sensitive subjects circuitously, Soa tended to approach such subjects, particularly those regarding her legitimate needs, very directly. When she needed money, she asked for it, with no excuses and no explanations. When one day, as I was leaving the village to go to the capital city of Antananarivo, she unexpectedly—and without pleasantries—handed me a list of the items she would need for her coming birth and baby. I took the list and did as she said, buying cotton, scissors, gauze, alcohol, hat, blanket, sweater. "Anything else?" I asked.

"No, that is what I need to have a baby," she answered, having expected me to provide all that she needed, but no more than that.

As Soa's pregnancy drew to a close, and she continued to work her *tavy* fields, Lita fell very ill. He lay by the fire in their small two-room home, and grew increasingly weak. Naina was called, and his diagnosis was as they feared. Lita had albumen.

Albumen is an indigenous classification for illness characterized by swelling feet, hands, abdomen and face; yellowing of the eyes, nails and palms of the hands, and darkened urine. People differ in their opinions regarding whether it is or is not accompanied by fever. Some suggest that the skin leaves a dent if pressed, and others point out that the *marary* (sick person) will sleep a lot and only eat greasy foods. They generally agree that it is an illness of older people, with some saying only older people can get it, and others saying that younger people can sometimes get it.

Its cause is not always agreed upon, though many say that it is caused by too much salt in the diet. Others say that it is brought on by becoming too cold, or by drinking too much *toaka*. Some say that it is caused by wind entering the body, which makes the body swell up. Others say that it is caused from eating too many sweets, while many say that it is caused from not having enough food. Soa echoed the sentiments of many when she said that it was usually inherited.

"If a person gets it when they are old, then it is inherited from their parents," Soa explained, "and if this happens, then all the children of the parents will get it when they grow old. Most old people do get it, there is much albumen in Madagascar. You cannot escape it. But if a young person gets albumen," she continued, becoming very sad, "then it is not inherited. If it is the first time the generation has had it, then it is contagious."

"Albumen?" Dr. Tovo, of the Park Project, explained, "albumen is something in the blood, it is a protein. What you are describing sounds more like *tazo vony*," he said, referring to what would be literally translated as "yellow fever," but which he translated as hepatitis.

"*Tazo vony* is not the same as albumen," Nirina explained to me, after I told her what the doctor had said, "*tazo vony* can turn into albumen, but there is no swelling with *tazo vony*. Only yellow skin and yellow eyes."

"And *tazo vony* will not kill you," Soa added, "it may linger, but it can be cured. The *ombiasa* can cure *tazo vony* but they cannot cure albumen. Not even the *doketara* [doctor] can cure albumen."

"No, the *doketara* have many medicines, but none to cure albumen," Nirina concurred. The women had stopped by my house for afternoon tea, which we were drinking outside in the rain, under the thatch awning of my cooking area.

"If the *ombiasa* and the *doketara* can do nothing for albumen, is there anything that the family can do? Are there forest medicines or other treatments?" I asked.

Soa answered. "Foods or medicines that bring on diarrhea sometimes help, because the abdomen is swollen with water and this makes the water leave. And if the illness is caught early, the *ombiasa* might be able to cure it, but the there must also be a *saotra* [ceremony of thanks to the ancestors]. If the *ombiasa* doesn't catch it early, it may be temporarily cured, but it will come back"

"What will happen to Lita?" I asked gently.

"He will die." Soa answered, matter of factly.

"Yes, *andriamanitra* [God] will take him," Nirina, schooled in Catholicism, concurred.

The women finished their tea by the fire and as Soa rose to pound rice for Rivo, Nirina announced that it was time to go home and bicker with Faly, her husband of half a century.

Despite the agreement that only the *ombiasa* could do anything, no matter how ineffective, to help the person suffering from albumen, how the healers themselves diagnosed and viewed the illness differed, even within the tiny village of Ranotsara. For example, Naina said that it could be cured, but if it was cured, it became *fefy*, another indigenous classification usually, but not always, used synonymously with *tazo vony*. It would never really go away, he explained, but remain dormant, ready to reappear at any time. Naina, an *ombiasa*, provided his own views on the cause and treatment of the disease.

"There is an egg in the heart which causes the hands and feet to swell. The reason I know this is because the sick person likes to eat a lot of eggs. When an egg remains in the body, the body needs eggs. It is *fady* [taboo] to eat meat and salt when you have albumen. When the egg is deprived of meat and salt, the person will vomit the egg."

"Have you ever seen this happen?" I asked, skeptically.

"*Eny ary* [oh, yes], I have seen it," he answered. "The egg is not in the shell. It is very, very young. *Angroso* is the name of the illness at this stage, when the person has vomited the egg. If the egg is not vomited, the *marary* will die. The illness will spread from the face to the hands and feet. The illness begins with the face and eyes turning yellow, and the urine is very dark. When the hands and feet become swollen, the illness has spread."

"How do you diagnose it?" I asked him.

"To diagnose it," he answered with considerable patience, "I look at the eyes, face and fingernails. If the person is *malemy-lemy* [sort of weak], does not respond to me, and their face, eyes and nails are yellow, I know that it is albumen."

"Do you consult the *sikidy?*" I asked, referring to the divination system commonly used to diagnose social and physical discord.

"No, I do not consult the *sikidy*, if I have seen the symptoms myself" he answered, "because I know albumen. But if the treatment does not succeed, I will consult the *sikidy* to ask if there is another treatment that may work."

Rakoto, on the other hand, a young but popular *ombiasa* in the village, and a distant cousin of Naina (both of the Zafinaraina lineage), said with pride that he could indeed cure albumen.

"Albumen is contagious, it is spread through sneezing," he told me. "It is also caused by eating too much sugar. To avoid it, eat bitter things."

"Who can get albumen?" I asked him.

"Anyone can get it, especially adults who don't eat enough bitter things. But it always begins with another illness that is often very different. That is why I consult the *sikidy*."

"How do you cure it?" I asked him, ready to note down the treatment.

"The treatment is never the same," he responded, "the ancestors will tell me how to cure it, through the *sikidy*."

Soa and her family called upon Naina to treat Lita. Knowing he could not cure the disease, they sought to alleviate his discomfort. Soa went to the fields to gather extra firewood to keep him warm through the night, and she killed most of her few chickens to boil and feed to him. The broth is believed to provide strength to the sick, and people try to maintain a stock of chickens for times of illness.

Lita grew progressively worse as Soa grew progressively bigger with her pregnancy. Her sadness became even more marked, and she spoke of the future as if his death would bring her the relief of caring for him, but with it would also come the uncertainty of her own future. Not owning any land of her own, it was only through her children that she could claim rights to the land, by farming it for them until they came of age. To return to her own village would be equally uncertain, as her brothers had been using her own land for so long that to claim it back (women having rights to one-third of all property from their parents) would cause family problems.

"I will ask Rivo if I can stay here," she said, "and he will let me, because I have nowhere else to go, and my children are the same as his own children. And I will sell my bananas to make the money to buy food and supplies for the next year."

Soa's *tavy* fields were planted with bananas, which she had been tending since my arrival. Aside from the wages she received from me and Rivo, she had no other assets to fall back on. But as the harvest season approached, Lita's illness grew critical, and she tended him night and day. Finally, knowing he would die at any time, but knowing as well that she had to get her bananas to market before they grew overripe, she returned to her fields with her children to assist in the harvest.

The bananas were gone. Every last one had been harvested. Only someone living nearby and knowing she was unable to tend the fields while Lita lay sick, could have stolen her bananas.

That night, before going home to help her husband die, Soa got very drunk. The next morning by five a.m., she was back at work, pounding rice for Rivo, raising the six foot pestle high in the air and bringing it down hard, again and again, as the pounding rhythm rocked her unborn child.

Death That No Medicine Could Prevent

Albumen is not, however, always regarded as an inherited or contagious illness. Even those who argued forcefully that albumen was a disease that was natural (coming with age), from the environment (brought with the weather), social (contagious), or brought by Zanahary [God] (a category including both genetic and environmental disease), found none of these explanations fully accounted for the illness of Faly, *mpanjaka* of the Zafindraraoto lineage.[3]

Faly appeared to be an old man, who guessed his own age to be somewhere between eighty and ninety, but it was probably closer to seventy. His grandfather, Ramanjato, was the founding member of the Zafindraraoto lineage, the alleged slave caste. He and Nirina, of the Zafinaraina

---

3. I was not present in the village when Faly fell ill, and the following account was drawn from interviews with those who treated and cared for him, as well as the ever-prevalent village gossip.

lineage, had been married for about fifty years, they guessed. They worked hard together, and they drank hard together. Laughing and joking endlessly, Faly never forgot his role as *mpanjaka*, taking the position very seriously. He lamented the changing status of his role, as poverty and limited labor led him to relinquish his fields to Rivo, and deaths and expenses forced him to sell his cattle one by one. By the time I arrived, Faly's status had diminished from that of a village leader, to that of an honored elder. The true leaders of the village, he suggested, were those who had no titles, but controlled the land.

In mid-November, Faly suddenly became very dizzy and feverish. He went inside his home to lie down, while Nirina nursed him. He had no appetite, and his eyes became very red. Soon, the tell-tale yellowish tinge that signals *tazo-vony* indicated that it was time to call for an *ombiasa*. Nirina sent for Rakoto, and he consulted the *sikidy*, learning from the ancestors that Faly was the victim of *mosavy* [witchcraft]. It did not take the family long to discover the likely *mpamosavy* [witch], as she was right there in the family — Faly's younger sister, Lanto.

In her mid-forties, Lanto was much younger than her elder brother Faly. Her isolated life as a single woman raising her children by herself, compounded by her inability to work her fields due to her poor health, contributed to her image as a social outcast. More importantly, she was rumored to be a thief.

"Rumors!?" Nirina spat out, "*Ny marana!!*" [the truth]. "I caught her stealing our bananas, our coffee, our sugar, even our chickens! They were no rumors. She was always stealing from us, and she finally stole so much that Faly did not have enough to eat. That was why he became sick, he was *hungry*. But he wouldn't do anything about it; he said she was his sister and she needed the food. *We* needed the food, too. So Faly and I got divorced." Nirina began to weep, thinking back to the terrible row they'd had that led her to storm out of their home and take up housekeeping in her adopted son's abandoned home.

"But I never stopped cooking for him, he still had to eat," she explained, reclaiming her pride.

Although their separation was a source of gossip and good humored fun in the village because everyone knew it would subside, once Faly became sick, Nirina moved back to their home. But neither her nursing, nor Rakoto's prayers and healing plants, could restore Faly's health. He grew sicker and sicker, and within two weeks, he was dead.

As I returned to the village following a brief absence, I saw Nirina awaiting me on the edge of the ricefields. She stood, rigidly erect, until I approached. Having heard the news of Faly's death, I greeted her with sadness and, breaking the Malagasy *fady* of never crying for the dead after their burial, Nirina fell in my arms sobbing. She'd lost her best friend.

Within weeks of his death she was working the rice fields alongside women a fifth her age. Nirina, whose age and ancestry marked her as the most respected and noble woman of the village, was working for Rivo.

Faly's death left the position of *mpanjaka* open for his younger brother, Kotomahay, to assume. Having recovered from the illness that fell him and his grandson, Solo, Kotomahay proudly accepted the office informally, and began acting the part of village leader, presiding over important decisions, welcoming guests, and joining the other *mpanjaka* in ceremonial duties. Until the weather cleared and the *sikidy* was consulted for an auspicious ceremonial date, the inauguration—in which a cow would be sacrificed, great quantities of *toaka* drunk, and everyone certain to be singing and dancing throughout the night—would have to wait.

"I am your father, now," Kotomahay told me upon my return to the village, "because I am taking Faly's place, and I will be as a father to you as he was a father to you while you live with us. Soon, when the deaths have stopped, I will move to his home. But for now, we must wait, because it is in his home that the dead of our lineage must be lain. And I am sorry to tell you that I have received news of another death. My niece has been living in a village far from here, with her husband and children. She died yesterday, of *tazo vony*. Because she grew up here and lived here until her marriage, her body will be brought back here so that she may be buried with the ancestors. But the village is far, and it will be another two days before her body arrives. After she is buried, if the deaths have stopped, I will move to the *trano be* [ceremonial house, used for funerals, and in some cases as a house of the *mpanjaka*]."

It rained sideways for the next two days, a cold and wet isolation, as the village turned into an island of mud. Talk began to circulate that if the *maty* [dead one] did not arrive soon, the river would rise so high it would be impossible to cross. And if the body did arrive, many wondered, would it even be possible to get it up the slippery hills to the tomb without dropping it altogether? No, it was agreed, this was no time to die.

But the river hadn't yet risen so high that the pallbearers couldn't cross it. After three days, the body was borne high on the shoulders of a group of men unknown to me. The residents gathered at the edge of the village to greet the *maty*, and murmurs immediately exploded in exclamations of surprise. The four days that had passed since her death, had caused her body to bloat beyond recognition; she resembled an obese pregnant woman, and I was assured that she was neither. The smell was so terribly fowl that even her closest friends expressed discomfort at sitting with the body, which soon oozed putrid body fluids onto *tsihy* after *tsihy* [grass mats, wrapped around the body].

"They can't keep that body here much longer," Bemaso complained on the second day, wrinkling his nose, "the whole village smells of *maty*."

"Why haven't they had the funeral?" I asked.

"Because her family must come from far away," he explained, "so we must wait. But I think they should just take it away right now, it's going to bring more death."

"Yes," Lalao agreed, "they want to wait for the family to arrive, and they must, because it is the *fomba*, but it has been too long. If it isn't taken to the tombs soon, then more death will come."

"How much longer will they wait?" I asked.

"Until tomorrow, *angamba* [maybe]?" Lalao asked, not sure of the answer herself.

Fortunately, the answer came soon, as the family and friends arrived, filling the mud-drenched village with the festivity of reunion and the sorrow of their loss. The funeral was held in the rain; as the body was brought out, the putrid grass mats were piled onto a clean grass mat for disposal in a sacred grove of distant trees. The mourners rushed toward the edge of the village to see the body off, where it would be taken to the caves deep within the protected forest and left to join the ancestors.

I stood under the tole awning of a two-story house, watching as one by one they left the *trano be*. When the village had emptied of any sign of life, with the mourners all gone to say good-bye to the dead, I was surprised to see one more mourner slowly leave the *trano be*, his head buried in his hands as he sobbed loudly at his loss. Kotomahay lifted his head and looked at me, slowly approaching. He spoke in a low, barely comprehensible mumble, not meeting my eyes.

"She was my brother's daughter, I raised her as my own. She was a happy child, always laughing. But *tazo vony* kills everyone, even the young. We have no medicine for it. The doctors have no medicine, the forest has no medicine. Only the ancestors know who will be next." He gazed at the *trano be*, the clay house he longed to make his home, yet the place of so much death. He slowly walked back and picked up the *tsyihy* tied into a bundle. It was growing dark and the rain was beginning to fall again, harder with each passing minute. Without a word he began the slow walk in the growing wet darkness to dispose of the bundle.

The next afternoon, the rain still coming down like hammers and nails, he approached me again as I made my rounds from house to house.

"The walk to the forest has been very hard on me. My head hurts and I feel dizzy. Do you have aspirin?"

I did, and I returned to my house and found some. He accepted gracefully and without comment, slipping into his home to rest by the cooking fire.

By nightfall he was in a coma.

The next morning visitors surrounded him as the *ombiasa* were called. Albumen, one said. *Tazo vony* another said. *Aretina biby*, they all said, when the truth was discovered. Kotomahay had not taken the bundle deep into the woods, it turned out. Instead, with the rain and darkness coming on, he had dropped it off in a sacred grove of trees, distant, but not distant enough, from the village. His niece's ghost had struck him ill to curse him for this *fady*. His final diagnoses, ghost sickness.

At the end of the day he was still unconscious. With the rains falling harder and harder and the winds picking up, getting him to Ranomafana was impossible, and viewed as pointless. Only the ghost of his niece could save Kotomahay, but there was no sign of mercy. As the night drew near midnight, the wind began to howl and the rain began to hammer the earth harder and harder. With a loud smack, the cyclone hit, sending sheets of tole flying, thatch roofs crashing, doors slamming open and shut. And at almost that very instant, the howling of mourners began. Just a few yards away from my own door, I barely discerned the loud wailing of the women that had grown so familiar a mark of death. The wind was so loud, the cyclone so fierce, that the wailing sounded far, far away. Pounding on my door, Colette burst in, drenched, babbling and flaying her arms.

"Another death!" she said, "hurry, come!"

We rushed out the door and through the rain slamming down in the pitch black night, expecting to find Lita dead, but finding instead twenty or thirty people crowded outside Kotomahay's door.

He would reach the *trano be* after all, but not as the resident *mpanjaka*, instead as the next *maty*, the fourteenth since I'd arrived, less than a year before.

Three days later, as Kotomahay's body was taken into the forest to join the ancestors awaiting him, the wailing began once more. Lita, whose illness had lingered for two months now, had passed away, as his wife readied to give birth.

As I returned home in the cyclone following Kotomahay's death, I found my home crowded with women from the Zafinaraina lineage. The cyclone, the midnight hour, the rapid succession of deaths, had all electrified the women, and amidst the shock and sadness there was an intoxicating buzz, as everyone chattered at once in efforts to explain how another death had hit so hard and suddenly. Lalao hurried to cut up some fruit and serve it to our guests as I stood around dazed, babbling expressions of shock and sorrow and fussing with a petrol lamp. Giving up, I lit a paraffin candle just as Lalao handed me a plate of pineapple and I sat down to the table, Colette, Soa, Lalao and others crowding around as if for a seance.

"Kotomahay's death was no accident," Colette whispered, slowly and clearly, as if speaking to a child, to be sure I understood. "He was *andevo*. His whole family is *andevo*. That is why they have all been dying." The wind and the women continued to wail in the darkness beyond the door, and the rain continued to batter the metal roof. Through all the unearthly whistling and wailing, we could barely hear the rapid pounding on the door, but we gradually turned our heads one by one as the beating became louder and more and more demanding. Lalao opened it and a small quick figure shrouded in a yellowed-plastic sheet slipped into the dark and tiny room. My little comrade, Toky, wasn't going to let this gathering take place without him. His dancing smile lit up the corner where he silently tucked himself, eyeing the pineapple like a starving Oliver Twist until Lalao passed him his share.

I voiced my confusion. "But Nety died, Tantely's son died, Baoroa's grandchild died, Ramasy died. Bao died. Your own children have died. They were not *andevo*, they were all Zafinaraina," I pointed out.

"Yes, but look at all the others who have died. Kotomahay, Faly, Tsaralahy, Solo's baby, Jenine, they were all *andevo*." Colette smiled smugly as if her reply had proven her point.

"Yes, Janezi," Toky interrupted, teasingly, from the dark corner where he crouched "*andevo*...," said as if to send a light-hearted chill up my spine, knowing it was a word I'd grown to know well, and therefore just the sound of the word would clarify it all.

I did not understand. I had been keeping track of the deaths, and they were nearly equally divided between the two lineages. I could not determine any common feature, aside from apparent malnutrition, high fevers, and the lack of health services. From my (layperson's) view, a few had died of hepatitis, a few children from malaria, two from malnutrition probably compounded by illness, a couple were just very old. But lineage, which did appear to play a roll in daily health care, seemed unconnected to the deaths. As Nirina had said, Tanala die, Betsileo die, Vazaha die. The same could be said for the Zafinaraina and the Zafindraraoto. The illnesses which killed hit all, while the illnesses which merely slowed and impaired hit hardest on the poorest. Colette's *andevo* explanation made no sense to me.

Soa interjected.

"They are cursed. The ancestors have sent death to them, and death to our village, because they have married too many among us." I thought of her own "royal" husband who lay dying as we spoke.

Colette could not keep quiet, she was bursting to disrespect the local "other." As always, Lalao stood quietly aside, cleaning up after us and taking note of the talk, to take back to her parents, Rivo and Kalamira.

"An *andriana* would never have done what Kotomahay did," Colette continued, "by leaving the *tsihy* among sacred trees. *That* is the act of an *andevo*." She sucked the juice from her pineapple as she ate it in a few rapid bites.

"But Kotomahay was a very good man," I protested, feeling uncomfortable that someone who I had found to be so warm and kind to me would be disparaged only moments after his death.

"He was a *great* man!" Colette countered at once, and everyone joined in praising him. It appeared that they could easily distinguish the man from the lineage, while the lineage remained inseparable from his identity. He was, according to this conversation, descended from slaves, thereby still colored with the stain of history, a stain that would linger through generations to come. The lineage explained his weaknesses, just as it explained their strengths, but individual strengths among the "*andevo*" Zafindraraoto and weaknesses among the "*andriana*" Zafinaraina were attributed to one's personal character. Prejudice looks the same wherever one finds it, I thought to myself, still uncertain how deaths among the Zafinaraina were explained.

The Birth of a "Tanala"

The night that Kotomahay's body was taken to the forest, a forest that a resident could legally enter only as a corpse, Lita died, and he, too, was carried away in the raining night to his own *andriana* forest tomb. A few weeks later, as I began to awaken to the familiar and surreal cries of lemurs in the nearby distance, Lalao burst into my room, urging me to hurry and awaken.

"Soa has had her baby," she said, handing me a cup of coffee she had roasted and pounded herself. Her tone was very sober.

"How is she?" I asked, concerned for Soa and disturbed that I'd slept through the event. I'd wanted to participate in a local birth, a desire Soa found odd but agreeable.

"There is a problem. The afterbirth has not come. The baby was born six hours ago. Soa is in much pain. They've sent for Alarobia's wife in Ambatovory. No one here has been able to help her."

I hurried to dress and rushed off with Lalao. Colette met us on behind the house.

"Soa told me to go get you, when the baby was coming" Colette said, "but I was afraid to wake you up. *Vazaha* like to sleep." Colette, for once, was serious.

"It's a girl," she added soberly, as we reached Soa's house.

The whole village had gathered outside and although no one was wailing, the mood was anxious and grave. We entered quickly, our heads bowed low.

Soa was huddled in a corner, the same corner in which her husband had died a few weeks before. Her mother, who had traveled from a distant village to assist her daughter, was beside her. Nirina and Kotomahay's wife, Soary, were assisting her. Nirina held Soa as Soary reached deep into Soa's uterus. Soa made no sound, just stared off to the side. A tiny baby wrapped in a soiled cloth lay next to her mother's legs, the cord still uncut. The baby made no sounds at all, but squirmed quietly and helplessly. Her head was already wearing the tiny knit hat Soa had asked me to bring back from the city. A baby must have its head covered at all times, no matter how hot, to keep it from getting *marikoditra*, a fever with chills.

No one seemed to notice the baby, it lay all alone beside Soa.

Just then, only moments after we'd entered, Baofaly, arrived. She was married to Alarobia, the *ombiasa* in Ambatovory, and was noted for her midwifery skills.

Wasting no time, the elderly woman directed Soary to give her a plate. Soary moved quickly and found an enamel plate, pouring water from a plastic cup into the shallow-sided plate. She carefully handed it to Baofaly, who dropped some leaves into the water, and offered it to Soa to drink. As Nirina helped Soa drink the herbal water, Baofaly reached into Soa's uterus as so many others had been doing for hours, and pressing on Soa's abdomen with one hand and twisting her arm inside the suffering woman, she expertly pulled out the afterbirth as Soa grimaced silently. As Baofaly placed the afterbirth on the grass mat, a heavy sigh and murmured thanks to Zanahary, the Christianized indigenous deity, filled the room, and then the baby was picked up.

The cord was cut and the dirty cloth quickly stripped from the baby, who was promptly dressed in her new acrylic knit clothes. Soa rested in continued silence by the fire, not looking at all to her new child. The women passed the baby from one to the other, each commenting on what a beautiful child she was, when finally Nirina, with great decorum and a somber face, handed the baby to me with the announcement, "Janezi, you are now Tanala."

And with that, the room burst into hilarity as I took the bundled child in my arms, and the door was opened to the crowd to gaze upon the new life.

A few months later, the baby, named Emma, died just as three of Soa's other children had in the last two years.

I recalled a picture Soa urged me to capture with my camera, late in her pregnancy. Snatching up a fat healthy baby of six months, Soa held it against her bulging belly.

"Take this picture, Janezi!" she called out to me when she saw me wandering around with my camera. "Tell the *vazaha* that we Tanala like having babies so much that we have another as soon as they're born!" And laughing in merriment at her perceptive joke, she handed the baby back to his mother, then picked up a six foot pestle to pound more rice for Rivo.

Chapter 9

Conclusion

In this ethnographic study of forest farmers in Madagascar, I set out to show how the use of medicines by indigenous people who live in the seemingly exotic realm of the rainforest extends beyond plant medicines and "traditional" medical beliefs. My concern has been, instead, to illuminate the multiple ways in which environmental and social changes penetrate indigenous knowledge systems in such as way as to create complex and ever-changing interplays between changing environments and access to health resources.

I have presented what I describe as a political ecology of health perspective to understand these complex relationships. Specifically, I suggest that the environmental and health nexus can be understood as a socially mediated process, in which local, national, and international policies and practices are interconnected, influencing one's health and relationship to the environment in differing ways. Rather than viewing environmental change as directly affecting the health of people in a given society in uniform ways, I contend that social and environmental changes affect people unevenly, and their health is thereby affected in multiple ways. Among the variables that shape these uneven relations, my analysis has focused on economic status, lineage, age, and gender as salient to the ways in which the changing forest landscape has influenced health practices and beliefs in one small village strategically located amidst an internationally-funded conservation and development project in southeastern Madagascar.

While my findings regarding the village of Ranotsara are unique to this village at this particular place and time, and unique in that they have been represented through the filter of my own subjective analysis, the village level study is particularly salient to a political ecology of health analysis because it shows how national and international policies and practices have very distinct implications at the local level. In the village of Ranotsara, a history of social tensions related to lineage and economic status have divided the village in such a way that it has been impossible for the community to experience the benefits or consequences of social and environmental change uniformly. Moreover, these pre-existing social fissures have deepened with recent conservation and development initiatives, and these social divides have had serious health consequences for some, but not all, residents of the village.

Three important points have been raised in this study. The first is that conservation of the forest has had adverse economic effects among forest residents, leading to less ability for the majority to purchase pharmaceutical medicines and greater neglect of chronic illnesses, rather than increasing reliance on plant medicines. The second is that contrary to the prevailing view that one's cultural or ethnic identity determines how they perceive and use their environment, and determines one's medical beliefs and practices, I found, instead, that just as concepts of the environment, and of health and healing in the United States are understood in terms of education, family income, and social power, so too do these same factors mediate one's understanding of, and interaction with, the environment and the medical realm of Ranotsara. The third point that I have presented is that current practices related to the forest and to health are not the stuff of tradition, but must be understood in historical and social contexts.

In what follows I elaborate on the evidence I have presented to support these points.

Forest Medicines

There remains a proclivity among educated Westerners to conceptualize forest medicines as botanical resources representing an ancient wisdom of that which is wild and untouched, offering potential remedies and cures to the pains of affliction. These ideas are not entirely off target. People living in the forest do, indeed, have extensive, if variable, knowledge bases of the potential medicines surrounding them, and there is no doubt that the botanical bounty of the tropical forests conceals potential medicines for many grave and debilitating illnesses.

But one's knowledge of the botanical inventory, and their use of these medicines in their daily lives, is influenced by age and gender. While there was a considerable diversity of knowledge about the local plant habitat in Ranotsara, I found that men and older women have a greater knowledge of the botanical inventory of the region than do younger mothers. This is, I believe, because Ranotsara is a patrilocal village, and the diversity of Madagascar is such that even within short distances, ecosystems change. As such, as young women marry and move to Ranotsara, they bring with them the botanical knowledge of a different region. In some cases, there may be considerable consistency in which plants are used, and how they are used, but in other cases, different plants might be used for different purposes. Women therefore exchange information about these medicines, leading to an ever-changing knowledge base among women as to which medicines to use for which illnesses. As women age, their knowledge of the local botany increases, and becomes more consistent with the knowledge of other elders, both male and female.

To pass on their knowledge, however, they often rely upon sons, because they will remain in the area as they grow into adulthood, while daughters are also taught the values of local medicines so that they may treat their own children. Thus, women's indigenous knowledge of plant medicines differs from men in that it is not just passed on generationally, but it is also passed on to others within generations.

This generational knowledge, however, is unlikely to be as "ancient" as one might presume. As I recounted in Chapter Six, the village is relatively recent, having been founded by two separate groups of people a century past. Thus, there have only been a handful of generations who have lived in the Ranomafana region, their ancestors having come from the highlands. Villagers' familiarity of the local botany therefore reflects not only the knowledge brought from these highlands, but also suggests new knowledge, as grandparents of the present inhabitants in all likelihood incorporated new plant species into their healing repertoire. Thus, it is likely that contemporary indigenous knowledge of healing plants is characterized by innovation and modification, consistent with Western science.

But at the same time that older people are indeed more knowledgeable of indigenous medicines than are younger people, they are also more accustomed to pharmaceutical medicines to treat illness. They have become, in many respects, habituated to the colonial health care system. Those who live in the forest do not live cut off from the rest of the world. The medical systems of indigenous societies are syncretic systems of healing, and as such, pharmaceutical medicines have been incorporated into local pharmacopeias as important and efficacious healing resources.

While pharmaceutical medicines have been cognitively and practically incorporated into indigenous medical systems, not everyone has access to them. The consolidation of economic power in Ranotsara has enabled certain village residents to maintain a ready supply of pharmaceutical medicines for treating respiratory disorders and fevers, while the rapid decline in economic status of most residents and the associated decline in their nutritional and health status, has contributed to a growing dependency upon forest and local indigenous medicines for others in treating these same illnesses, though they are more likely to seek treatment only when these illnesses become acute or interfere with their work or other responsibilities.

Nonetheless, despite the ability of certain men and their families to access health services in Ranomafana and elsewhere—services which are appallingly inadequate and likely in many cases to worsen one's health—the poverty of everyone, combined with an unhealthy environment, extremely demanding work loads and geographical isolation, have contributed to poor health for all village residents.

Among the narratives I presented to support this point, the story of Nety's death is particularly demonstrative. Nety had died from an apparent seizure at the river's edge, and although her death prompted numerous and conflicting explanations, the physician's concern that she had stopped taking her seizure medication because she could no longer afford the medication, is persuasive. Nety was of the more noble Zafinaraina lineage, which conferred upon her a higher social status than her Zafindraraoto counterparts, and provided her with important and close ties to those who controlled the majority of land and resources in the village. But as a landless, unmarried mother, her gender and youth countered any benefit her lineage bestowed upon her, and her ethnicity failed to account for the fact that her illness had not been treated. The neglect of her illness was not necessarily from ignorance, but may have been from her having become accustomed to the efficacious properties of the pharmaceutical anti-seizure medication. It is conceivable that plant medicines would not be used as a substitute, because they were not regarded as efficacious for the treatment of a seizure disorder.

A second example I presented to support my point that illness is suffered by all and that pharmaceutical medicines are integral to the healing repertoire though often unavailable, is the story of Lanto. Lanto, whose story I presented in Chapter Seven, was from a lineage reputed to be descended from slaves. Her lineage, combined with her status as an unmarried, middle-aged woman, rendered her a social outcast, despite being the sister to her lineage's *mpanjaka*. Her lineage, gender, and marginality in the community contributed to minimal social support in maintaining her fields and restoring her health. Her poverty thus exacerbated, her lack of access to medicine, health care, and knowledge contributed to her chronic illness. Her ethnic identity, whether imposed or self-identified, seemed to have little bearing on the treatment strategies she pursued; she herself showed little faith in the healing faculties of Rakoto, who, like all the *ombiasa* of Ranotsara and nearby, was of the Zafinaraina lineage. Instead, she neglected her illness until persuaded by the physician to seek biomedical care; her repeated and futile efforts to do so eventually exhausted her, and she returned to her customary treatment, neglect of her illness most days, *ahibalala* tea when her condition worsened.

The neglect of her illness was not necessarily from her ignorance; the stories of chronic illness which I have presented illustrate the way that discomfort and illness have been naturalized by many who, although not necessarily regarding themselves as "healthy," have surrendered to the futility of trying to combat so many health concerns, a futility Lanto came to know well.

The incorporation of pharmaceutical medicines into African healing systems has received attention from others who have shown the ways in which the steadfast belief in African "traditions" is slow to recognize that African practices are generally based on reasoning and experience, rather than superstition and ignorance. For example, Vaughan (1991) has shown how even as colonialists recognized the rapid acceptance of pharmaceutical medicines in eastern Africa, they continued to explain the incorporation of biomedicine into indigenous healing systems as evidence of Africans' continued belief in 'magic;' the colonialists presumed that the Africans interpreted the efficacy of biomedical drugs as magical, and not "scientific." On the contrary, as Feierman (1985) has indicated, Africans do practice biomedicine and do become educated as Western-trained physicians. The incorporation of biomedicine into indigenous African societies is indeed an African practice. It is misleading, also, to suggest that as Africans become educated in biomedicine that they cease being African, or that indigenous medicine remains the backward practice of rural Africans uneducated in Western science (Feierman 1985). Such a conception is generally promoted as rooted in cultural tradition and tied to ethnicity.

Culture, Ethnicity, and Medicine

A second, and perhaps the most important, point which I have made in this study is that the use of medicine and of the environment is not related to one's unchanging ethnic identity, but is instead more closely associated with one's lineage, education, and social status, as well as access to land and labor. Moreover, policies which presume that health and environmental perceptions and practices have ethnic origins, are potentially harmful.

In the story of Solo and Kotomahay's illnesses, and that of Solo's malnourished son, which I presented in Chapter Eight, I explained how I found myself drawing on my own prejudices to explain the neglect of the baby's nourishment to ignorance, which struck me to be in stark contrast to the attention Solo's aches and pains received. While I focused on what I perceived to be ignorance, a failure of people to recognize the severity of malnutrition as compared to a common flu, the people of the community focused on one's relationship to the forest, or how one is, or is not, empowered to control the land and resources of the forest that surrounds them. As economic power diminished for nearly everyone, families came to rely more on the power of the ancestors to remedy social problems, not because they were bound by traditions and unable to understand the severity of malnutrition, but because they viewed themselves as relatively powerless in the changing community and therefore drew on the most potent power they felt that they could summon.

To some, however, the illness and death in this family might have been understood in terms of an alleged "Tanala" ethnic identity, while the differing approach to the sickness and death of Jeanine's baby might be conceptualized in terms of her family's declared "Betsileo" ancestry. But to distinguish the differing illness strategies as reflecting differing ethnic views of medicine would be misleading because it would obscure the ways in which poverty and local kinship ties have mediated the illness experience for these families. I found their different economic positions, accompanied by different familial ties, to be more salient to understanding how one explains and treats illness in Ranotsara than is a focus on ethnic difference.

Another example which I used to show how ethnicity does not directly relate to one's use of medicines was in the story of Celine and Zanabelo. Celine and Zanabelo consulted Zanabelo's cousin, an *ombiasa*, regarding illnesses of their children, and I suggest that their decision to do so had more to do with their trust in someone from their own lineage than it did solely in their belief in his magical powers. Lineage, alone, however, could not explain their actions, as they handled each illness episode in their family differently. They sought Western medicines when they were affordable and available, used indigenous plant medicines when the illness was deemed ordinary and treatable, and sought intervention of the *ombiasa* when the illness was believed serious but unnatural, with cosmological origins. Thus, multiple factors influence their treatment strategies and cannot be easily reduced to either lineage or ethnicity.

Nonetheless, lineage has had considerable bearing on one's economic power, which in turn influences health. To understand this relationship of lineage to economic and health status, as well as to how one interacts with the environment, it is necessary to contextualize present practices and beliefs in the social history of the region.

Historicizing Health and Environmental Practice

The third point which I have emphasized in this study is that in order to understand how local social relations relate to health and environmental practice, it is necessary to understand local and national histories. As political ecologists have shown, land use is not the simplified process of continuing degradation promoted by many policy-makers. It is uneven, both temporally and geographically. Moreover, land use change is not necessarily perceived as degradation by inhabitants of the forest; those who live in or near the forests of what is now the Ranomafana National Park view the land in terms of its productivity and subsistence value, regarding the earth as more valuable than the trees which grow on it.

In Chapter Four I discussed the history of pre-colonial and colonial policies regarding land reorganization in Madagascar in order to show how forests are conceptualized and used by contemporary people on the island. I argued that the pre-colonial autocracy and colonial government shaped land and resource use through social policies including forced labor, taxation, relocation, conservation, and development. Understanding this historical context helps to understand that concepts of "traditional" land tenure regimes, as I also demonstrated for "traditional" medicine, and "traditional" cultural identities, have been anything but "traditional." Moreover, the most severe environmental degradation in Madagascar, attributed to "Tanala" farming methods, is actually more closely related to Madagascar's urban industrialization. Industrialization of the Merina empire, combined with social and land reorganization, fostered massive deforestation and concentrated people in the most forested areas. This deforestation was further exacerbated as colonial forest policies divided one million hectares of forest land into nine separate reserves and redefined these areas as "protected" areas. In so doing, the prohibition of *tavy* was linked to the enclosure of forests for conservation purposes, at the same time that exploitation of these same forests was facilitated by laws regulating and sanctioning the use of the forest for industrial development. The portrayal of *tavy* as environmentally destructive was perceived as contradictory by forest farmers who saw that the trees and plants of the forests were viewed as resources of value to outsiders. As such, they remained dubious that conserving the forests was intended to benefit them in any way, or that the forests would not eventually be depleted anyway.

In Chapter Five I discussed how the history of land reorganization and agricultural policy has been specifically tied to changing identities. In particular, I focused on the history of Merina, Betsileo and Tanala ethnic identities. The Ranomafana National Park Project used "cultural sensitivity" in much the same way as colonialists throughout Africa engaged in "indirect rule," to persuade residents to adopt new practices. In so doing, they reified social differences as ethnic ones, ranking the ethnic groups in terms of their modernity.

The cleavages produced by land reorganization in the nineteenth and early twentieth century were further exacerbated by post-colonial processes and events, including structural adjustment, land privatization, the Gulf War, and cyclones. These events, combined with unequal distribution of project benefits, enabled a few families to consolidate their land and resources, and appropriate the land and labor of their more disadvantaged neighbors and kin. The ensuing economic inequality, however, was due as well to existing social divisions in the village; these same processes have had different consequences in different parts of the region, a distinction which illuminates, rather than refutes, the significance of integrating international and national policies and processes with local-level processes.

The consolidation of economic power in Ranotsara has enabled certain village residents to maintain a ready supply of pharmaceutical medicines for treating respiratory disorders and fevers, while the rapid decline in economic status of most residents, and the associated decline in their nutritional and health status, has contributed to a growing dependency upon forest and local indigenous medicines for others in treating these same illnesses.

The current agricultural system employed by subsistence farmers in Ranotsara combines *tavy* with irrigated rice agriculture and cash crop production. Rather than representing three different types of agricultural systems, as treated in project policy, the land is farmed as a single system in which three different cropping strategies are practiced simultaneously to maximize yields. In Ranotsara, the majority of farmers where I lived owned *tavy* fields exclusively, lacking the labor and suitable land for irrigated rice, while a minority owned (or rented from others) irrigated rice fields. Most all had some sort of cash crop land, such as bananas or coffee.

With the declining economy of many families, and their greater workload as they labored, like Soa, Solo, and Lanto, on their own and others' fields, illnesses intensified. While all families suffered the experience of one or more early deaths, the prevalence of illness was greatest among those who lacked sufficient nutrition, and were unable to treat their illnesses in a timely manner because they lacked the money for medicines.

While the concept of the ICDP's, or Integrated Conservation and Development Projects, has now been abandoned in Madagascar in favor of a regional focus, in which conservation and development initiatives are tailored to specific regional needs, the regional focus remains problematic because national conservation policies, as well as development initiatives, must remain in accord with international environmental policies if nations are to continue receiving financial support from international donors. Given the history of colonialism and post-colonial policies that produced such profound social dislocation and impoverishment throughout many parts of the world, along with the current trend toward globalization of a capitalist economy, national policies related to resource use and the economy are unlikely to operate in isolation from transnational interests.

International concerns have made environmental protection a priority for many of the world's leaders, who have tied the use of environmental resources to economic objectives. The alliance of environmental concerns to economic ones is not without merit. But when environmental concerns are divorced from issues of environmental justice—that is, a focus on how the most subordinated groups disproportionately suffer from environmental degradation or contamination—and further divorced from issues of social justice—a concern for the equitable distribution of material and social resources—then environmental policies all too easily become socially legitimated forms of social control. In order to understand how it is that this can happen, it is worthwhile to consider how environmental policies are socially constructed.

The Use and Misuse of Science in Conceptualizing the Environment

The language of global environmental management has been crafted in such a way as to make a focus on the historical and cultural contexts of environmental change impossible to incorporate into international policy. Hildyard (1993) shows how the United Nations Conference on Environment and Development (UNCED), held in Rio de Janeiro in 1992 and popularly regarded as the Earth Summit, framed the environmental crisis in terms which concealed the role of the North in creating the crisis, while casting the North as the only possible solution to the problem. For example, he notes that environmental problems were consistently stripped of their history by divorcing contemporary problems from the past. References to 'recent,' 'new,' and 'the latest' data suggested that environmental problems are something new, and in the Earth Summit, these problems were presented by 'government,' 'international' or 'industrial' authorities, thereby safeguarding the credibility of those whose actions have historically produced contemporary environmental problems.

Hildyard further indicates that by treating environmental problems as 'global' problems, no one in power is held responsible for creating them, and to the extent that responsibility is suggested, it is in terms of a 'lack of knowledge,' with all of humanity having a shared stake in the survival of the planet. In this way, too, the authority of the North was legitimated by the UNCED in the humane call to save the planet.

> Few environmentalists would argue that environmental degradation has reached critical proportions—destroying local livelihoods, condemning species to extinction, blighting landscapes, and (if climatic disruption occurs on the scale predicted by some climatologists) possibly threatening the very future survival of humans and other mammals. But within UNCED the critical nature of such threats was used to justify giving those currently in power still more authority; to legitimize programs which would remove control still further from local people; and to sanction more management, more top-down development, more policing and still greater control of people (Hildyard 1993:31).

The use of language to construct diverging and paradoxical worlds permeates the debates among researchers trained in varying methods, theories, and concerns, and among administrators charged with carrying out the national and international agendas of global ecology. These differing languages also reflect a fundamental discord distancing social scientists from policy makers. The discord between social science and conservation/development (for the two are very often interchangeable in the globalized era), runs deep. In many cases this divide is characterized as an academic divide, in which the social and the biological sciences are portrayed as dueling disciplines, with social scientists speaking an unintelligible language and failing to recognize the environmental crisis confronting the planet.

This disciplinary divide was expressed in a recent e-mail exchange regarding conservation and development issues in Madagascar, but could be extended to any geographical locale where institutional economic and social changes are targeted toward indigenous communities. In April of 1997, David Meyers, Program Officer for the International Conservation of Tropical Environments (ICTE) at the State University of New York at Stony Brook, solicited feedback from researchers regarding a proposed consortium for research and training in Madagascar. Publishing his appeal on *Hevitra*, an e-mail list-serve for scholars of Madagascar, he suggested that the failure of social scientists and physical scientists to engage in productive discourse was impeding the objectives of conservation and development. In reply, Professor Maurice Bloch suggested that such an appeal did not reflect a genuine interest in cooperation.

> I am wary because in my previous experiences of this matter I have found natural scientists deliberately avoiding the work of the social scientists who, like myself, have worked in Madagascar, and found them trying to replace it by their own "social scientists" whose research is usually superficial but more amenable to their aims and thinking. The reason is that what we have to say is too difficult and too much of a challenge to their ideas and that, as [historian Edgar] Krebs says, natural scientists lack the historical and cultural perspective which would explain to them 1) that for Malagasy peasants conservation is but one new and very similar manifestation of interference and bullying by the outside (which to them includes the Malagasy state). 2) Ideas about conservation are a very new, very historically specific, fad in the West which is difficult to impose [and] at great cost on others [and] as though it was based on eternal truths. Natural scientists never hear that message, not only because they don't want to, but also because since they are ALWAYS seen as government agents they are treated by the Malagasy peasants with justifiable fear ... and so with agreement and endorsement in the hopes that they will go away.

It seems to me that the problem in the proposed consortium is that the interests of the Malagasy concerned and of the natural scientists are fundamentally opposed and so, if social scientists represent and explain what the Malagasy feel and think, they too, will be opposed to what the conservationists want. Before plunging into a joint enterprise genuine, really genuine, dialogue must take place. It will be most upsetting to all. (Maurice Bloch, April 3, 1997, Research and Training in Madagascar, emphasis his. Available e-mail Hevitra-L@psuvm.psu.edu)

In reply, Meyers thanked the author for his comments and urged "all who are interested to contact the World Bank, USAID, and other large donors for the most recent documents on the PE2 [Second Environmental Program of Madagascar] for further clarification." (David Meyers, April 3, 1997, Research and Training in Madagascar. Available e-mail Hevitra-L@psuvm.psu.edu). He further suggested that environmental programs were, in fact, established and implemented by Malagasy institutions, implying that the *Association National des Gestations et Areas Protegee* (ANGAP) [National Association for the Management of Protected Areas] and other national institutions, which are funded wholly or in large part by U.S. and European monies, are not under control of Westerners, but are instead, the national institutions they purport to be.

A response to Meyers pointed to the fallacy of his reply.

Although not out of character with the record in these matters, it is still dismaying that an invitation to bring together in a consortium the very real concerns of biologists and social scientists doing work in Madagascar could be followed so speedily by a different sort of invitation, i.e., to carry those same concerns to the World Bank, USAID, ANGAP, ONE, ANAE and DEF.... Charging at windmills and having a conversation with colleagues are not the same thing. None of the points raised by Dr. Bloch and by myself were addressed in David Meyers' response. He just passed them on.

The notion that the Malagasy are the driving force behind ANGAP and that the Second Environmental Program (PE2)— "The Landscape Approach"—comes straight from the Sakalava, Betsileo, Vezo, Tandroy, Tanosy, Antemoro, Antambahoaka, Anatefasy, Masikoro, Betsimisaraka, Zafimaniry, Tanala, Mikea, Antakarana, Mahafaly, Bara, Tsimihety, Tsihanaka, Merina and (why not) Vazimba...sounds a bit disingenuous to me. Perhaps it is the suspension of belief needed to accept or go along with all this—more than any horrible disciplinary divide—that stops conversation (Edgar Krebs, April 4, 1997, Research and Training in Madagascar, available e-mail Hevitra-L@psuvm.psu.edu).

Krebs' response itself stopped the conversation. There was no further interest expressed from Meyers or others, at least none that reached the *Hevitra* list-serve of Malagasy scholars, regarding bringing together social and natural scientists.

Despite the very real divide which separates the sciences, this divide is conjured to obscure a much greater, and far reaching, divide, and that is the one which severs social science from conservation and development policy altogether. While conservation and development policy is economic policy, which would imply a commitment to social science, in their application to environmental concerns policy makers have relied upon the biological sciences to legitimate their agendas. By prioritizing the science of the physical world over the study of the social, they have couched the dialogue in the language of the biological sciences. But it is a dialogue they know not well. As Krebs asserted,

> The majority of conservationists I met while doing fieldwork in Madagascar knew very little of biology. . . . Biologists should also be concerned that of all the USAID money earmarked for conservation in Madagascar, only an invisible percentage has gone to fund research. I regret that there are no long-term studies of the ethology and ecology of lemurs comparable to those made by Jane Goodall on chimpanzees; no studies of the ecology of the Malagasy forests comparable to those conducted by Charles Elton in the woods of suburban Oxford; no literature on Malagasy birds that can match the essays by W.H. Hudson in "Birds of La Plata." This underlying ignorance of the natural history of Madagascar justifies the perception many Malagasy have of international NGO's operating in the island. Quoting Alex de Waal, "they see not people who are making a sacrifice to assist the poor and vulnerable, but immensely rich foreigners who descend from aircraft (and 4-wheel drives) spending a short time consulting with local people, never in the vernacular." ("International NGO's and Complex Political Emergencies: Perspectives from Anthropology," Royal Anthropological Institute, London, 1995:10) . . . The creation of a consortium is not necessary if one is aware of the problems attending development/conservation projects (in Madagascar and elsewhere), of the literature they have generated and that otherwise bears on them (which is already a rich conversation in many disciplines), and—more pointedly—of the work ethnographers and historians have done and are doing right now in the island. (Edgar

Krebs, April 3, 1997, Research and Training in Madagascar, available e-mail Hevitra-L@psuvm.psu.edu).

Krebs points to a very real concern in the application of science to policy, and that is that while relying upon the biological sciences to legitimate their objectives, conservation and development administrators are, by and large, generally ignorant of science, or of the possibilities that exist for enhancing both research and policy by actually reading the work that is generated by researchers of all persuasions. For example, the very nature of research in the natural sciences has brought such researchers in day-to-day contact with local residents, who are employed by them as guides, cooks, and interpreters. Moreover, natural scientists are *researchers* and as such, most have an appreciation for the research process, regardless of its disciplinary foundations. In my own experience, the natural scientists conducting research in the Ranomafana National Park were much more concerned with the social ramifications of conservation policy than were the policy makers themselves, in part because they spoke to residents and saw for themselves the chronic poverty of the region. In addition, they generally showed intellectual curiosity in the work of social scientists. While there remained a definite and discernible distinction between the language and objectives of social and physical scientists (with those of the physical scientists far and away more central to the objectives and concerns of policy makers), discussion between researchers was frequent and in many ways fruitful, as each informed the other of important data and perspectives which enriched both realms of research.

But Krebs raises the issue regarding the use of the biological sciences to legitimate policy and promote the idea that it is the inability of researchers to communicate, rather than the unwillingness of administrators to incorporate the concerns of researchers into ready-set economic agendas, that renders conservation and development projects ineffective and potentially destructive of local societies and lives.

> Casting such a reaction in terms of an academic divide, of that lazy misnomer: paradigm problems; or of an essential quarrel between the social sciences and biology, is rather perverse. It is shifting the ground and looking at another scene not to look at what is happening before our very eyes, which is perfectly straightforward and easy to read. If the tables were turned, anybody, biologists included, would be horrified at the sight of a "native" marking off and rearranging our backyards to suit wholly alien criteria. And any biologist (I would if I were one) should equally balk at the sight of a nebulous field, implicating her/him and his/her profession, a field which slides from biology to conservation to development in erratic ways,

ones certainly not governed by the ethics inherent to the pursuit of knowledge (Edgar Krebs, April 3, 1997, Research and Training in Madagascar, available e-mail Hevitra-L@psuvm.psu.edu).

Indeed, it was my experience that conservation and development policies were implemented in Madagascar with little or no regard for the rights of human subjects. Whereas researchers are required through their institutional and professional associations to abide by clearly specified codes of conduct, no such code of conduct exists by which development or conservation planners must execute their policies. Lacking any agreed-upon code of ethics, conservation and development administrators may well be led to invoke a morality of "science" in the pursuit of economic change.

Global Patterns of Conservation

Protected areas comprise close to ten percent of the Earth's surface (McNeely and Scherr 2001). But these protected areas are not devoid of people. Over one billion people, or approximately one-fifth of the world's population, live in the 25 biodiversity "hotspots" of the world.

At least 16 of the 25 biodiversity hotspots are located in areas with very high malnutrition; they encompass fully one quarter of all the undernourished people in the developing world. Countries that include biodiversity hotspots and in which more than a fifth of their total population is undernourished include: India, Nepal, Thailand, Laos, Cambodia, the Philippines, Papua New Guinea, Democratic Republic of Congo, Republic of Congo, Kenya, Madagascar, Namibia, Cameroon, Bolivia, Haiti, Dominican Republic, Honduras, and Nicaragua. Under-nutrition rates in several large countries—including Mexico, Guatemala, Brazil, Peru, Ecuador, China, Indonesia, and Vietnam—are much higher in the vicinity of biodiversity hot spots than for the country as a whole (McNeely and Scherr 2001:8).

These figures suggest that the stories of illness and malnutrition presented in this book are anything but rare. Indeed, poverty, poor health, and malnutrition are more the rule than the exception for those people living in protected areas of the world. Nonetheless, this poverty is accompanied by increasing concentrations of wealth for others, a point not missed on McNeely and Scherr (2001:9) who note: "At the same time, increased concentration of wealth has meant that fighting obesity and other problems of excess food consumption is now a preoccupation in Western countries and among urban elites in developing countries." As the world increasingly depends upon the market economy to solve all its problems, including health and environmental concerns, economic stratification intensifies, and along with it, as some people profit, other people lose land, homes, and livelihoods. Understanding international environmental policy thus requires understanding its ideological underpinnings and how these ideologies are related to economic and political objectives. These objectives shape and inform the scientific process by which relationships between humans and their environments are understood.

While the Ranomafana National Park and the story I have related of my experience living in the park region suggests a unique and disquieting history of poor planning and ineffectual policies, the Ranomafana National Park and the USAID project that supported it, reflect current environmental views and policies that have contributed to processes of social dislocation and economic stratification throughout the world.

For example, Neuman (1998) has argued that the national park model which characterizes protected areas throughout the world was fashioned after Yellowstone National Park. Yellowstone was created at the turn of the twentieth century as a place for the upper-middle class to escape to, a recreational landscape free of the stresses of urban life (Chase 1986). This objective required the eradication of those species which were, or were perceived to be, threats to humans. Wolves were systematically slaughtered, bears intentionally starved to death, and bison eliminated. Only those species deemed enjoyable were permitted to survive. In some cases, species were introduced, such as trout for the enjoyment of fishermen. The results of systematically eliminating some species, while introducing exotic species, were ecologically profound, and resulted in erratic environmental policies, as well as decades long suppression of any scientific research which might bring to light problems with the strategies and objectives of the park (Chase 1986).

Moreover, Chase argues that in order to achieve the restful utopia Yellowstone's creators envisioned, it was necessary to eradicate the history of Native Americans from the land. This was done by denying the role of Native Americans in setting fires which facilitated new growth and promoted agriculture, and by denying their role in hunting certain species, sometimes to extinction. By revising history to suggest that Native Americans never played a significant role in the Yellowstone region, the concept of the ecosystem as pristine and untouched by humans prior to settlement by whites was reified; in other words, it became possible to argue that there was a "natural" state which could be preserved for the enjoyment of visitors. This historical revisionism was compatible with both racist views of Native Americans as "uncivilized" (because they were not credited with the agricultural sophistication of understanding the role of fire in agricultural production), and with more sensitive perspectives that recognized the horrendous atrocities committed against the native peoples (by denying their role in hunting and thereby reducing or eradicating species, native peoples were viewed as inherently protective of nature) (Chase 1986).

Conserving nature is a relatively new objective of national parks. Neumann (1998) argues that the concept of parks existing to preserve the native ecology was a secondary goal to early conservation movements, whose primary objectives were to safeguard landscapes for the pleasure of those who could afford to travel to them. It is only in recent years, he suggests, that the ecological objective has become the primary objective. Nonetheless, he suggests that tourism is fast becoming the world's largest industry, leading to a revival of the turn-of-the-century thinking of parks as centers of consumption. Thus, the idea of parks as serving the aesthetic ideals of Anglo-Americans remains central to policy and management decisions of national parks today (Neumann 1998).

As this park model was transferred to Africa during the onset of colonial rule, similar social views of indigenous peoples as separate from the environment shaped land policies. For Europeans during the nineteenth century, Europe was viewed as that which was cultural; Africa was their countryside, their nature. Those living within it were regarded as features of the landscape, but not as active fashioners of the landscape. The history of Africans, then, was removed from the history of the world, just as the native peoples of North America were removed from its history. Africans, as conceived by the conservationists who established national parks throughout the continent, had no history—they were frozen in time, viewed as primitive fossils. Even today, much academic discourse centers on pre-colonial, colonial, and post-colonial periods; in many of these representations, the precolonial is either represented as utopic and egalitarian, or uncivilized and ignorant. In both cases, the precolonial period is viewed as unchanging.

Neumann (1998) further shows how most of the land that is now enclosed as protected areas or national parks throughout Africa, was established from lands which had been appropriated by the colonial state. This land, once appropriated, was often used for big game reserves, in order to ensure a steady supply of big game for the British elite to hunt. In other cases, the land was appropriated for use as settler estates, such as plantations on which Africans were forced, directly or indirectly, to labor for the profits of the Europeans. In either case, Africans have been excluded from the parks, except to the extent that they are compatible with images of Africans as primitive, savage, and animal-like. By making Africans a part of the landscape, and savage at that, they became dehumanized as part of the fauna of the landscape — they, too, were a part of the wildlife. And those Africans who did not behave like primitive Africans, could not remain in the park (Neuman 1986). It is not surprising, then, that national parks are not well received by those who live within or adjacent to them. Perceived as a continuation of colonial policies of land and resource appropriation, along with social engineering, the national parks which appear to many tourists as scenic wonders to be preserved, strike many others as something entirely different.

National parks increasingly depend upon ecotourism not only to bring in money, but also to increase public acceptance of their role. Along with the ecotourism that is fast becoming a profitable industry tied to conservation, comes ethnotourism, designed in large part to mitigate the social consequences of such environmental engineering. Ethnotourism attracts tourists concerned with the growing homogenization of cultures, as indigenous practices and belief systems rapidly give way to the cultural trappings of the Western world. Despite concern for maintaining cultural integrity and survival of the world's most marginalized peoples, too often ethnotourists are confronted with — and expect to find — the very stereotypes conservationists of the colonial period created to promote protected areas in the early twentieth century, such as displaying indigenous peoples as frozen in time, revealing bare skin adorned with local grasses and bits of bone, and clutching spears or bows. Such imagery is picturesque and fits well with the undomesticated landscape of national parks.

The image of indigenous peoples as integral to images of the untamed wild runs, oddly, hand-in-hand with the image of indigenous people as destroyers of biodiversity. It is precisely indigenous interaction with the land that is pointed to as a chief cause of species depletion. As argued throughout this book, such an image is divorced from not only history, but from broader social factors shaping differential access to resources. But a question remains, is it not necessary to preserve certain areas of the world in order to save them, even if this means that "these people" will have to accept changes in their lifestyle? Aside from the obvious response, which is to suggest that lifestyle change be demanded of all the world's people, rather than only those most poor and powerless, it is necessary to consider whether protected areas actually serve their purpose. In other words, even if they fail at any social objective, such as increasing incomes, maximizing agricultural efficiency, and slowing population growth, do they achieve their environmental objectives of preserving species diversity and ecosystem integrity?

As Chase (1986) has shown for Yellowstone, by tenaciously clinging to the idea that what they were doing was virtuous and unassailable, park administrators made it impossible for any real biological assessments to be made. Moreover, by assuming their policies were ecologically sound, there was no room for admitting mistakes. The result was that in their efforts to get Yellowstone back to its mythic primordial past, policy makers allowed the ecology of the area to be severely degraded as species were endangered or eliminated, and exotic species thrived.

Similarly, Vandermeer and Perfecto (1995) suggest that environmental destruction often remains invisible, particularly when it is tied to the changing global economy. Specifically, they point out that environmental protection is closely tied to the global economy, and associated with increased international trade. Such trade inevitably leads to an increased use of resources. Those resources that are consumed may not be in "preserved" environments, but instead, take the form of increased use of fuel, toxic waste, pesticides, garbage, and an increased demand for renewable and non-renewable resources, all of which are associated with the manufacturing and marketing of products for use by consumers in the world's wealthier countries.

This increased production, along with the increasing poverty of indigenous people who have lost access to their lands and resources, contributes to profound ecological destruction, while "islands" of "wilderness" are preserved (Vandermeer and Perfecto 1995). In other words, the focus on conservation reserves or parks, when not linked to broader economic issues, leads to protection of *spots*, and increased environmental degradation beyond these spots.

Moreover, McNeely and Scherr (2001:3) report that

> Protected areas inevitably lose species when surrounded by landscapes that bring alien invasive species, pollution, and development pressure. According to projections based on accepted ecological principles, if only the currently protected land areas remain as wildlife habitat, between 30 and 50 percent of the species will still be lost, because the reserves do not contain populations large enough to maintain the species.

Thus, not only have protected areas had profound consequences for the health and well-being of the world's poor, they have also failed to achieve their honorable goal of preserving ecological habitats, largely because they have emerged from concepts of nature as separate from people, and in so doing, have created artificial zones of paradise for tourists and scientists to savor, for the good of the world.

In Closing:
Culture and Ethnicity
Applied to Policy

In presenting these intersections of health and environmental change, it becomes apparent that forest medicines, and forest health, can only be understood in the context of forest lives, a context which has thus far been essentially excluded from policies related to health and the environment. The exclusion of a social context—as fundamental to policy, rather than as a component to it—may be due to the sad reality that human lives have not received the public attention that the lives of endangered species have received in seemingly exotic places such as Madagascar. While considerable attention (both scientific and popular) is drawn toward the plight of Madagascar's lemurs[1] there has been scant attention drawn to the health effects that material and environmental changes have caused the Malagasy people. But the Malagasy people, like people everywhere, are divided by their own internal divisions, arising from shared and diverging histories, environments, communities, and economies.

By showing how these internal divisions have contributed to how one uses the forest environment, and in turn, mediated the illness experience, I have sought to challenge prevailing views that the relationship between health and the environment can be understood as a causal one, in which tropical environments have predictable effects on human health. I have also sought to dispel notions that a "cultural context" is something that can be interjected into such a causal relationship in a simplified manner that conflates culture with race or ethnicity. The political ecology of health approach I have employed has emphasized the internal divisions of the community in shaping the interactive relationship between health and the environment.

The Ranomafana National Park Project legitimated its social control of the region through the idea that biodiversity is threatened, it must be preserved, and the best way to preserve it is by providing economic alternatives to residents. To support and facilitate this objective, it sponsored an endless stream of scientific researchers seeking to catalog and observe the

---

1. In addition to the plethora of PBS specials and natural science magazines devoted to the endangered flora and fauna of the island, witness such titles as "Infant Death in Propithecus diadema edwardsi at Vatoharanana, RNPP, Madagascar" (Erhart 1997) "Effects of Food Availability and Forest Composition on Feeding Patterns of Propithecus diadema edwardsi" (Hemingway 1996), and "Psychological Well-Being of Nocturnal Primates in Captivity" (Wright, et al. 1989).

non-human biological species of the region. But by using science to legitimate health, land, and agricultural policies, the Ranomafana National Park Project recast social tensions, inequalities, and competing power interests as cultural traditions in need of technological remedy. And while doing so under the cloak of cultural sensitivity, they elicited sets of "cultural beliefs" from questionnaires that, as Millard (1992:4) has indicated to be a common practice among health professionals, ended up trivializing the relationship between cultural systems and health. In the case of the RNPP, the relationship between health and the environment thereby became one in which practices and beliefs were sorted into one of two "cultures" and so sorted, equated with one of two "agricultural systems" that allegedly held differing "threats" to the environment, and consequently justified social regulation.

In associating cultural practices with agricultural systems, the project conflated culture with ethnicity, presuming that ethnic identity and cultural practices were the same thing. Having it fixed in their minds that the "Betsileo" and the "Tanala" represent two separate identities and, most importantly, two separate "cultures," project reports began to reify the distinction by indicating that the cultural system in which the project was launched was characterized by two distinct groups, the "Betsileo," whom they claimed are more amenable to social change, and the "Tanala," whom they characterized as clinging tenaciously to their traditional practices (RNPP 1994). Because the project viewed environmental change as something that is fundamentally wrong and its social impact uniformly experienced by local residents, it was unable to explore the ways in which local residents used their environments to maintain their health and standard of living, and more importantly, how the social structure in which residents lived differentially influenced how they would use the local environment. Hence, environmental change was conceptualized as "forest exploitation," "deforestation," or "slash-and-burn" farming, and culture was reduced to ethnic affiliations in which "Betsileo" were positively evaluated, while "Tanala" were negatively evaluated. It was no wonder, then, that when the project established a local ethnographic museum aimed at increasing tourists' cultural awareness, the museum was adorned with photos of hard-working irrigated rice agriculturalists identified as "Betsileo," and music-playing, dancing, singing, shaman-worshiping, forest-burning "Tanala."

The project tied these ethnic distinctions to health by employing a Malthusian model of population increase to explain the relationship between health and environmental change (RNPP 1994). Primary health care was regarded by Project officials as necessary for three reasons. First, increased population pressure was identified as the primary threat to sustainable conservation efforts. Second, improving people's health was reported as essential to maintaining economic productivity of the local population. And third, because the residents identified health care as their most important need, providing it was regarded as good P.R.

Because those identified as "Betsileo" were regarded as more intelligent and more amenable to change, they were consequently viewed as more likely to adopt family planning practices. Those identified as "Tanala," in contrast, were not only regarded as less healthy than "Betsileo" — their poor health was regarded as their own doing, because they did not live like Westerners, did not have latrines, did not so readily join the globalized economy, and were viewed as culturally crippled in their own health care by their reliance on shamans over physicians. They were also regarded as being less likely to practice family planning. The actual beliefs and practices of villagers, which vary more on the basis of age, class, lineage, and religion, were ignored in favor of concepts of ethnomedicine that were essentialized in terms of ethnicity.

While employing the concept of ethnicity is often essential to understanding social identity, the use of the concept to gain an understanding of people's views and behaviors may block inquiry into other important cultural features which divide and unite people. The question remains, when applying anthropological concepts of culture to social policies, how do we draw out the more subtle and complex dimensions of identity which shape how people actively manage their environments and health? Anthropologist Kay Milton (1996) proposes reformulating the concept of culture to reach these interlocking dimensions of identity and social difference. She suggests thinking of culture in terms of what is unseen, that is, exploring how people's experiences shape the way that they think, interpret, and feel about the world in which they live. Whether such a definition draws us closer to culture or further from it (toward the individual, whose experiences take on cultural relevance through social discourse) is not so important as is the terribly obvious, but obviously overlooked, idea that people be asked about their experiences, feelings, and ideas about their world, before presupposing any cultural or "ethnic" traditions displacing such personal experience. When linking environmental change to changing health, it is these nuanced details of identity that draw us closer to understanding how the views and behaviors of differing groups of people forge the social and environmental linkage.

Contrary to the simplification of the local residents of the Ranomafana region as "traditional" people from one of two cultural groups, they are no different from people elsewhere in that they are active, contribute to the creation of their own cultures, and their actions and views are directly related to their social positions. Moreover, while these social positions do not *determine* one's actions or perceptions, they are influential, intersecting with personal experience. As Milton (1996) suggests, personal experience plays a salient role in the social construction of culture, and an exploration of individual experiences and narratives provides a telling portrait of cultural complexity. Nonetheless, one must be cautious that in so doing, the voice of the individual not be separated from the culture which has formed it through the production and reproduction of shared meanings, beliefs, and ideals.

Internal divisions have profound implications for social and environmental policy and projects but without exploring these divisions or incorporating them into project strategies, objectives to stop forest destruction will fail. In order to achieve the environmental objectives of USAID and the Malagasy government, for example, a better understanding of ethnicity and lineage is necessary. Such an understanding of social identity and its consequences, however, brings into question the morality of these environmental objectives when they are tied to social identity.

In the case of the Ranomafana National Park Project, while the project did not create the poor health in the region, nor cause the deaths of so many people, I would argue that the policies they established exacerbated the poor health in the region by limiting the economic options of the majority of residents, deepening social inequalities and divisions, and refusing to accept any responsibility for health, while at the same time they promoted an image to the public, to funding agencies, and to residents, that they did indeed provide significant health care to residents. Moreover, by being blind to cultural features outside the exotic realm of shamanism and slash-and-burn, they were unable to explore any possible relationship between the economic and environmental changes in the region and declining health. As a result, health care remained unavailable to some of the sickest human residents of the forest, while broader understandings of how health and the environment are intertwined differently for different social groups, remain elusive concepts to many environmental planners effecting social change.

The Ranomafana National Park was created from admirable objectives of safeguarding the planet and preserving life. Yet at the same time, in so doing, it affirmed hierarchies and values regarding whose life was worth protecting. This conservation ethic replicates the early eighteenth century construction of "wilderness" as a sublime and sacred landscape, a meaning which, by the nineteenth century, led to the necessity of taming the natural world for human habitation. By heralding the beauty of wilderness, a place inhabited by God, it became a spectacle for tourists to behold (Cronon 1996:12).

Cronon (1996:14) points to the irony of how it was the elite businessmen of the industrial age, those who had benefitted the most from the industrialization of America and its associated destruction of the environment, who most championed the wilderness as a domain of recreation, for "sleeping under the stars...and living off the land."

Thus, the decades following the Civil War saw more and more of the nation's wealthiest citizens seeking out wilderness for themselves.... Wilderness suddenly emerged as the landscape of choice for elite tourists, who brought with them strikingly urban ideas of the countryside through which they traveled. For them, wild land was not a site for productive labor and not a permanent home; rather, it was a place of recreation. One went to the wilderness not as a producer but as a consumer, hiring guides and other backcountry residents who could serve as romantic surrogates for the rough riders and hunters of the frontier if one was willing to overlook their new status as employees and servants of the rich.

In just this way, wilderness came to embody the national frontier myth, standing for the wild freedom of America's past and seeming to represent a highly attractive natural alternative to the ugly artificiality of modern civilization. The irony, of course, was that in the process wilderness came to reflect the very civilization its devotees sought to escape. Ever since the nineteenth century, celebrating wilderness has been an activity mainly for well-to-do city folks. Country people generally know far too much about working the land to regard *un*worked land as their ideal. In contrast, elite urban tourists and wealthy sportsmen project their leisure-time frontier fantasies onto the American landscape and so created wilderness in their own image (Cronon 1996:14, emphasis in the original).

If anything regarding wilderness has been conserved over the last two hundred years it has been this Western construction of the concept itself, as a landscape to be preserved for the fulfillment of those living far from it. The only significant change has been that technological advances have enabled many more people to travel to "remote" landscapes in search of "the primitive," in both landscape and society. Thus, not only does the taming of wilderness persist, so, too, do the processes of colonial control over land as the ever-expanding power of the world's wealthiest nations over post-colonial nations grows ever greater.

There is irony, too, in the fact that the very conservationists who have sought lifestyles and careers aimed at "getting back to nature" and escaping the stress of "civilization" by going to the far reaches of Madagascar, call for forest residents to leave nature alone and step up their own "civilization." Prohibited from transgressing the Maginot line of the Park boundaries, forest residents are separated from the forest, while ecotourists and natural scientists are ushered in, a process that also parallels Cronon's (1996) observations regarding the creation of U.S. national parks and the exclusion of Native Americans.

The myth of the wilderness as "virgin," uninhabited land had always been especially cruel when seen from the perspective of the Indians who had once called that land home. Now they were forced to move elsewhere, with the result that tourists could safely enjoy the illusion that they were seeing their nation in its pristine, original state, in the new morning of God's own creation. Among the things that most marked the new national parks as reflecting a post-frontier consciousness was the relative absence of human violence within their boundaries. The actual frontier had often been a place of conflict, in which the invaders and invaded fought for control of land and resources. Once set aside within the fixed and carefully policed boundaries of the modern bureaucratic state, the wilderness lost its savage image and became safe: a place more of reverie than of revulsion or fear. Meanwhile, its original inhabitants were kept out by dint of force, their earlier uses of the land redefined as inappropriate or even illegal (Cronon 1996:15).

Replicating this process of removing history from national parks to provide comfort for tourists, the history of the southeastern forests of Madagascar as sites of resistance and rebellion has been replaced with a history of primatology and soil erosion. At the same time, the contradiction of coercing residents into "modernization" in order that tourists and conservationists may enjoy the pleasures of escaping the modern world, is equally obscured. Perhaps this contradiction is best represented by the Project Manager's dream of an organic café in Ranomafana, where carrot cake and herbal teas made from local organic produce would be served to weary, hungry tourists. Those serving them would be the forest farmers who have farmed organically for centuries, now pushed to add chemicals to their own crops, and restricted to an economic system that is unlikely to enrich them, so that they might afford a piece of this wholesome cake for themselves.

Epilogue

One Last Death

My fieldwork came to an end in the same way as it began, with another death. On the morning of my departure, I awoke once more, not to the eerie cries of the lemurs, which had so enchanted my mornings and nights, but to the ghostly cries of women wailing for the dead. Mialy, a young woman in her early twenties, had died in the night.

Following eighteen months in the Ranomafana region and fourteen months in the village, I was summoned to the offices of USAID on May 10, 1996, and informed that the Ranomafana National Park Project, and the health component of the project, were irrelevant to my research. As such, I was advised to abandon any thoughts of including the project in my analysis of health and environment in the Ranomafana region, and particularly cautioned that I should avoid expressing any criticism of the project. I was further cautioned at the conclusion of this meeting that if I went "public" with my criticisms against the project, future researchers would be hurt as a result.

One month later, on June 4, 1996, I was summoned to the capital city of Antananarivo, for a meeting with two Malagasy officers of the *Association Nationale pour la Gestation des Aires Protegees* (ANGAP, funded by World Bank and USAID) and with three American representatives of the Ranomafana National Park.[1] Following a patronizing speech about the value of my research into "medicinal plants," I was asked to respond to a series of accusations levied against me regarding "the style" of my research, which they implied was potentially offensive to the Malagasy people.[2] More specifically, each member present, except for myself, was in

---

1. These representatives included the Malagasy Director General of ANGAP, a Malagasy woman who was not identified to me, the American Principal Investigator of the RNPP, the American Project Manager, and the American Conservation Director.

2. Pursuant to the United States Mutual Educational and Cultural Exchange Act of 1961, "no award granted by the Fulbright Board may be revoked or diminished on account of the political views expressed by the recipient or on account of any scholarly or

possession of a file that I was told contained testimonials that had been obtained in the course of an investigation that had been conducted in Ranomafana among people with whom I had worked with or had known, including waiters, hotel managers, acquaintances, tourists, project employees, local residents, and my research assistants. This investigation, I was told (Principal Investigator, personal communication, June 4, 1996), was not directed by the Malagasy, but was instead conducted under the direction of the American administrators of the project. When I requested a copy of the file, I was told that I could not see it, because it would reveal the identities of their sources. When I requested that they tell me specifically what the charges were, I was told that this information would also reveal the identify of their sources, and so I was not told of any specific charges. Consequently, I refused to respond to their request that I defend myself against unspecified charges by anonymous accusers.

When I would not participate in what I perceived to be an inquisition mimicking one that had been launched against a sociologist who had come under scrutiny of project administrators in 1993, I was pressured to leave by project officials who asked me to sign an agreement that I would not speak to anyone affiliated with the project in the absence of their supervisors, including the project physician and health staff, and that I would not express any of my "personal or philosophical views" to residents of Ranotsara. This secret investigation into my character and the unprecedented "agreement" that was presented to me, developed shortly after I began to seek healthcare records for the region to assess whether the high morbidity of Ranotsara was a new or unique phenomenon in the region, and as I became increasingly outspoken regarding my concerns for the health of local people. The document was handed to me by the American Project Manager. Written in French, it bore no indication of its origin—it was not printed on project letterhead, and it had no names other than my own. In essence, it was a document for which no one held responsibility.

The Principal Investigator silently awaited my response to her Project Manager's direction that I sign the document or, the American administrator

---

artistic activity that would be subject to the protection or academic and artistic freedom normally observed in universities in the United States. The Fulbright Board shall ensure that the academic and artistic freedoms of all persons receiving grants are protected." Culturally offensive behavior, however, can lead to the revocation of a research award. As such, as a Fulbright scholar, my personal view was that the focus on my alleged actions as potentially "offensive" was intended to facilitate my removal from the research project in a manner which would not lead to charges of suppression of academic research. That the sociologist who had been similarly charged with offending the sensibilities of the Malagasy was herself a Fulbright scholar, and therefore protected under the guidelines for academic freedom of the Fulbright board, also contributed to this view.

informed me, the government of Madagascar would revoke my research clearance. The Malagasy administrators present remained silent.

I had already been subjected to persistent and invasive inquiries into my views, behaviors, and habits by project officials. I was vaguely aware that project officials were questioning local residents about me, but I was unaware of the scope of the investigation, nor that it included the solicitation of signed testimonials. My mail had been delivered to the local post office and picked up, according to postal employees, by project employees. I received none of this mail. An envelope marked "confidential" which had been sent to me from the American Embassy arrived, having been torn open and re-taped. The letter bore the sad news that my father had died; the following day, having kept the news to myself, project employees I met on the road told me they were sorry to hear that my father had died. Having been offered the opportunity to leave my laptop computer at the project office, it was returned with a message that there had been unsuccessful attempts to crack the password. When I brought these practices to the attention of USAID administrators at a meeting of May 10, 1996, I was informed that such practices were not only acceptable, but that if I "attack the project or engage in an evaluation of the healthcare component, the project administrators will have a right to defend themselves" (field notes, taken during meeting with USAID administrators, May 10, 1996). Defensive action on the part of the project, however, was not based on informed discussion and the sharing of information. My experience was that it was limited to character assassination.

As such, by the time I sat down with the project administrators who had steadfastly refused to discuss the issues of health and environmental change which they seemingly "sponsored," I was unwilling to engage in further discourse because, just as with the project itself, the discourse of the meeting was far from participatory. It was, instead, a discourse orchestrated by those who sought to suppress meaningful dialogue in favor of maintaining an image of social and environmental responsibility.

Looking around the table to a group more divided in interests and objectives than those with whom I had been living the past year, but who shared the common agenda of preserving their jobs, I expressed my deep regret that the focus of the project inquiry became my personal and philosophical views, rather than the findings of my research which suggested that the conservation and development strategies of their project, in conjunction with local, national, and international economic and environmental changes, were contributing to alarming health problems.

To have agreed to not express my views to Malagasy residents would have not only limited my freedom of expression, but it also would have put me in the position of withholding information from the people with whom I was working. In short, it would mean that I not disclose to them the theoretical premise of my research nor the reasons for my questions. Moreover, because I perceived project employees, particularly members of the health team, to be subjects of my research, to refuse to speak with them in confidence and only in the presence of their supervisors, would have further violated the university contract I had signed concerning protecting the anonymity of human subjects. Although I raised these concerns to the people present, including the Principal Investigator, I felt that they showed no interest in, nor understanding of, the rights of human subjects.[3] Finally, I pointed out that by soliciting such information from members of the community in which I was conducting my research, the project eroded the relationships I had worked hard to establish in the community, thereby making it impossible to continue research in an open and honest manner.

Following the meeting, the Principal Investigator asked me to meet with her in private, during which time she expressed immense sympathy for my departure (apparently having forgotten her tacit acquiescence to the project's coercive tactics ensuring my departure and her refusal to share with me the contents of the file she retained regarding the investigation against me). Continuing to refuse to disclose any information regarding the "testimonials," she asked when I would be leaving. I indicated to her that I would leave the village within two days. As I reached Ranomafana, on my return to the village, I met someone at a hotel who asked if I were the person from Ranotsara. Indicating that I was, she said,

"It is really wonderful what the project is doing there."

"What do you mean?" I asked, surprised by the remark.

"Bringing them medicines, to help all the people who have been dying."

I had thought, by that time, that no actions of project administrators could stun me, but this statement certainly did.

"I didn't know about it. Who is bringing medicines?"

"[The Principal Investigator]. She is having Air Mad fly in Medicines. They will arrive Thursday. The doctor will take them out there."

Consequently, I remained in the village a day beyond my stated date of departure.

---

3. The ethical issues raised by the role of anthropologists working in or near a development project are complex. As Stewart and Strathern (2000) have discussed, with more and more anthropologists accepting employment as consultants, they find themselves increasingly divided in their loyalties to their employers and the subjects of their research, as well as increasingly constrained in what they publish. It is not uncommon, they indicate, for those who employ anthropologists as consultants to contractually restrict rights of publication. In this way, those who employ the anthropologist may prevent publication of anything deemed critical of the employer, and what is published, if anything, may be exempt from peer review and scholarly debate (Stewart and Strathern 2000:6).

Just as the woman at the hotel had disclosed, Dr. Tovo arrived the day after I was to have departed. He was bearing boxes of medicines. My suspicions as to the objectives of the project in dispensing medicines on the day after I was to have departed were betrayed in my face. Keeping his distance from me, the doctor made his introductions to the community. After some time had passed, I approached him in the presence of several community elders and leaders, and asked where the medicines had come from.

"They are not from the project, but the project has asked me to distribute them." He did not say, but it was clearly evident, that by having the project doctor dispense them, that they would appear to be providing them.

"Then where did they come from?"

"Air Mad, and Farmad," he answered. Air Madagascar is the national airline, while Farmad is a national pharmaceutical company, which produces low-cost generic forms of essential medicines. His answer sounded as if he were avoiding the question—Farmad may have produced them, Air Mad may have flown them in, but who provided them?

"I don't understand," I asked, "Who is behind this?"

He smiled, acknowledging my impatience and knowing well the frustration I had felt throughout the last year.

"A tourist was here when Tantely's son died. After you told her about all the people who had died, she went to Air Mad and Farmad and got them to contribute the medicines."

I felt like a fool. I remembered the tourist well, a Belgian woman who had come with a tour guide, hiking through the "primitive" terrain of the rainforest. She was one of the very few who passed through who showed any interest in the people. She came out of the house in which she was staying to find out what the wailing was about, and I, in my growing disgust with the indifference of my compatriots, remarked that this death was only one in a series, and I told her of my frustrated efforts at doing anything about it.

She apparently did something, something so simple, that I in my self-absorbed fury at the project's failure to act, had not even thought to do myself. She asked the people of Madagascar to do something, to provide essential medicines.

Of course, the medicines the doctor dispensed would do little to help in the long-term, and the health crisis in Ranotsara reflects similar patterns of health problems throughout the island. But the *act* of providing the healing substances would go far. And the people of Ranotsara knew well that it was not the project which provided the medicines, nor myself, but the kindness of a stranger passing through.

That night, as we boiled a pig to celebrate my departure, Tantely's sister grew ill. Only a few days before I had photographed her hacking away the rice in her brother's *tavy* fields, her cheeks swelling with the broad smile she displayed for the camera. Now, like Nety, and without warning, she began seizing. Dr. Tovo left the festivities to look over her. Administering anti-seizure medication, she promptly vomited it up. As the seizures grew more severe, he ordered some young men to hurry over the mountains to Ranomafana to get medicine he could inject.

As the hours passed and the villagers grew more and more intoxicated and well-fed, the music played and the people danced, the family of Mialy remained inside, anxious for the return of the young men. Dr. Tovo continued to try, futilely, to get the woman to keep the medicine down.

By nightfall the young men returned, half drunk, with no medicine. They told the doctor that the pharmacy was out of stock.

"They probably only went as far as Moratoky," he said, shaking his head and showing his frustration at his inability to help, and his profound sadness at the knowledge of what such powerful seizures would do to such a young and vibrant woman.

"But even if they went to Ranomafana, the medicine probably would not be there. There is not much medicine in stock," he conceded.

We pondered ways that he could keep the medicine down. He tried to push tubing down her throat, but it would not work. He deliberated ways to crush the medicine and inject it safely, but that idea would not work. In the end, there was nothing he could do, despite his boxes and boxes of Western medicine.

The village was too remote, the pharmacies too poorly stocked.

She died in the night.

And so my stay in the village ended with one last trip to the *trano be*, the "big house," which I had come to know as the House of the Dead. Expressing my sadness to her mother, a woman younger than myself, I left the village, having distributed my "essential" cultural objects to the hoards who surrounded me, in their hopes that I would bless them with the riches of the Western world, and their knowledge that I would not.

Genealogy Chart

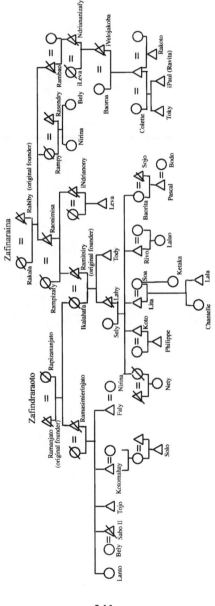

Glossary

ahibalala
Malagasy plant used to treat a multitude of disorders, primarily chronic coughs, colds and other respiratory illnesses

ala
forest

ala be
"great forest" or old growth

albumen
indigenous classification for illness characterized by swelling feet, hands, abdomen and face; yellowing of eyes, nails and palms of the hands and darkened urine. May be hepatitis, but diagnostic criteria vary by region and indigenous diagnostician. May be used interchangeably with *fefy* and *tazo vony.*

andevo
slaves or descendants of slaves

andevo fotsy
"white" slaves, similar to indentured servants who could buy their way out of servitude

andevo mainty
"black" slaves, formerly prohibited from marrying outside their caste or from owning land

andriana
nobles by birthright

angady
long-handled spade

ANGAP
Association National des Gestations et Areas Protegee - National Association for the Management of Protected Areas

an-tsaha
in the countryside; a term used in Ranotsara to refer to temporarily working distant fields

apanga
plant used to bring back the soul

aretina biby
ghost sickness

bay
boils, carbuncles and other skin eruptions

biby
ghosts

bilo
a form of spirit possession or ghost sickness; varies regionally

colons
colonial officers

corvee labor
unremunerated labor owed to the colonial state

Departement d'Eau et Forets
[DEF] Department of Water and Forests

doketara
physician

fady
prohibition or taboo

fanafody
medicine

fanafody gasy
indigenous medicine

fanafody vazaha
pharmaceutical medicine

fanompoana
forced labor during precolonial Merina rule

farasisa
wide range of subcutaneous skin disorders

faritany
province

fefy
indigenous classification for hepatitis-like symptoms; may or may not be hepatitis; sometimes used interchangeably with *albumen* and *tazo vony*

fehivava
land given in payment of a debt

firenana
lineage

fivondronana
sub-province; local political seat

fokonolona
line of descent arising from the same ancestor

fomba
custom

hantana
scabies

hazomanga
sacred wood

hetra
taxes; formerly collective property of the *fokonolona*

hibohibo
fallow land in later stage of growth than *jinja*

hova
free people

jinja
fallow land in early stage of growth

kabary
historical oratory

kabosy
home-crafted string instrument

kamo
lazy

katry
indigenous diagnostic category for fevers and seizures that affect small children

kidea
skin disorder; alleged to have been name formerly given to scabies

kitay
fuel wood

kohaka
cough

lamba
Malagasy cloth, often used as a shawl or burial shroud

laoka
any type of sauce with, or accompaniment to, rice

lolombintany
land granted by a royal chief or sovereign for services rendered

mainty
emancipated slaves or descendants of *hova* who had been reduced to slavery

maloto
dirty

marary
sick person

marikoditra
fever with chills

mosavy
witchcraft

mpamboly
farmer

mpamosavy
witch

mpandrary
jawbone from a cow used for weaving grass mats and clothing

mpanjaka
lineage leader

mpanjaka be
lineage leader of highest rank

mpitan-kazomanga
guardian of the sacred wood

mpitan-tranobe
　guardian of the big house

ombiasa
　indigenous healer or shaman

paraky
　tobacco

pirogue
　bamboo raft; canoe

sakay
　chile peppers

sempotra
　respiratory problems

sikidy
　divination system introduced by Arab traders during 15th century

taloha
　in the past, before

tamo tamo
　wild ginger root

tanana
　community, town, people

tanindrazana
　patrimonial land transmitted by succession or inheritance

tanim-bary
　irrigated rice field

tanim-pirenara
　lands divided into six states under Andrianampoinimerina

tavy
　swidden ("slash and burn") rice production

taxi-brousse
　privately-owned automobile used for long-distance public transportation

tazo
　fever

tazo vony
　literally "yellow fever" but may be hepatitis; often used interchange-
　ably with *albumen* and *fefy*

terres lavavolo
  vacant land

tety
  distant place

toaka gasy
  home-brewed alcohol, made from fermented sugar-cane

trano be
  ceremonial house, used for funerals; in some cases, it is the home of the *mpanjaka*

tsihy
  grass mats; used for many purposes, including wrapping the dead

vary lena
  watery rice

vazaha
  foreigner

Zanahary
  God

Bibliography

Abu-Lughod, Lila
1991   Writing Against Culture. In Recapturing Anthropology: Working in the Present. Edited by Richard G. Fox. Pp. 137-162. Santa Fe: School of American Research Press.

Alcorn, Janis B.
1995   The Scope and Aims of Ethnobotany in a Developing World. In Ethnobotany: Evolution of a Discipline. Richard Evans Schultes and Siri von Reis, Eds., pp. 23-39. Portland, Oregon: Dioscorides Press.

Allen, Philip M.
1995   Madagascar: Conflicts of Authority in the Great Island. Boulder: Westview Press.

Andriambelomiadana, Rochel
1992   *Librealisme et Developpement a Madagascar*. Antananarivo: Foi et Justice.

Antananarivo Annual
1898   The Population of Imerina and Measures for Increasing It. VI:247-248.

Archer, Robert
1978   *Madagascar Depuis 1972: La Marche d'une Revolution*. Paris: Harmattan.

Astuti, Rita
1995   People of the Sea: Identity and Descent Among the Vezo of Madagascar. Cambridge: Cambridge University Press.

Avotri, Joyce Yaa and Vivienne Walters
1999   "You Just Look at Our Work and See if You Have Any Freedom on Earth": Ghanaian Women's Accounts of Their Work and Health. Social Science and Medicine 48:1123-1133.

Baer, Hans A.
1982   On the Political Economy of Health. Medical Anthropology Newsletter 14(1):1-2,13-17.

Baer, Hans A., Ed.
1996   Critical Biocultural Approaches in Medical Anthropology: A Dialogue. Special Issue of Medical Anthropology Quarterly 10:4.

Baer, Hans A., Singer, Merrill, and Ida Susser
1997   Medical Anthropology and the World System: A Critical Perspective. Westport and London: Bergin and Garvey.

Banks, Marcus
1996   Ethnicity: Anthropological Constructions. London and New York: Routledge.

Barth, Fredrik
1969   Ethnic Groups and Boundaries: The Social Organization of Culture Difference. Bergen and Oslo.

Beaujard, Philippe
1983   *Princes et Paysans: Les Tanala de l'Ikongo: un Espace Social du Sud-Est de Madagascar*. Paris: Editions L'Harmattan.

Berthier, Hughes
1930   *Droit Civil Malgache*. Antananarivo: Imprimerie Officielle.

Blaikie, Piers
1989   Environment and Access to Resources in Africa. Africa 59:1:18-40.

Blaikie, Piers and Harold Brookfield
1987   Land Degradation and Society. Methuen: London.

Bloch, Maurice
1995   People Into Places: Zafimaniry Concepts of Clarity. In The Anthropology of Landscape: Perspectives on Place and Space. Eric Hirsch and M. Hanlon, Eds. Oxford: Oxford University Press.

1989   Ritual, History and Power: Selected Papers in Anthropology. London and Atlantic Highlands: The Athlone Press.

1986   From Blessing to Violence: History and Ideology in the Circumcision Ritual of the Merina of Madagascar. Cambridge: Cambridge University Press.

Bohlen, Janet Trowbridge
1993   For the Wild Places: Profiles in Conservation. Washington, D.C.: Island Press.

Boiteau, Pierre
1982   *Contribution a l'Histoire de la Nation Malgache*. Antananarivo: *Editions Sociales*.

Bryant, Raymond L.
1992   Political Ecology: An Emerging Research Agenda in Third-World Studies. Political Geography 11:12-36.

Bryant, Raymond L. and Sinead Bailey
1997   Third World Political Ecology. London and New York: Routledge.

Cameron, Mary M.
1996   Biodiversity and Medicinal Plants in Nepal: Involving Untouchables in Conservation and Development. Human Organization 55:1:84-92.

Campbell, Gwyn R.
1985   The Role of the London Missionary Society in the Rise of the Merina Empire 1810-1861 (A Contribution to the Economic History of Madagascar). Swansea: University College.

1992   Crisis of Faith and Colonial Conquest: The Impact of Famine and Disease in Late Nineteenth-Century Madagascar. *Cahiers d'Etudes Africaines* 127:XXXII-3:409-453.

Chambers, Robert
1983   Rural Development: Putting the Last First. New York: Longman Scientific and Technical, co-published with John Wiley & Sons.

Chase, Alston
1986   Playing God in Yellowstone: The Destruction of America's First National Park. San Diego: Harcourt Brace.

Collins, Jane L.
1991   Women and the Environment: Social Reproduction and Sustainable Development. In Women and International Development Annual, Volume II. Edited by Rita S. Gallin and Anne Ferguson. Pp. 33-58. Boulder: Westview Press.

Comaroff, Jean
1983   The Defectiveness of Symbols or the Symbols of Defectiveness? On the Cultural Analysis of Medical Systems. Culture, Medicine and Psychiatry 7:3-20.

Compte, Jean
1963   *Les Communes Malgaches*. Antananarivo: *Editions de la Librairie de Madagascar*.

Cousins, William E.
1895   Madagascar in the Year 1840. Antananarivo Annual V:342-344.

Covell, Maureen
1987   Madagascar: Politics, Economics and Society. London and New York: Frances Pinter.

Croll, Elisabeth and David Parkin
1992   Anthropology, the Environment and Development. In Bush Base: Forest Farm. Culture, Environment and Development. Elisabeth Croll and David Parkin, Editors, pp. 3-10. London and New York: Routledge.

Cronon, William
1996   The Trouble with Wilderness or, Getting Back to the Wrong Nature. Environmental History 1:4:6-19.

David, Thomas (J. Michael Beasley, translator)
1997   Miracle Medicines of the Rainforest: A Doctor's Revolutionary Work with Cancer and AIDS Patients. Rochester: Healing Arts Press.

Davis, E. Wade
1985   The Serpent and the Rainbow. New York: Simon and Schuster.

1995   Ethnobotany: An Old Practice, A New Discipline. In Ethnobotany: Evolution of a Discipline. Richard Evans Schultes and Siri von Reis, Eds., pp. 40-51. Portland, Oregon: Dioscorides Press.

Dubois, S. J.
1938   Monographie des Betsileo (Madagascar). Paris: Institut d'Ethnologie.

Durrell, Gerald
1992   The Aye-Aye and I: A Rescue Journey to Save One of the World's Most Intriguing Creatures From Extinction. New York: Simon and Schuster.

Ennis-McMillen, Michael C.
2001   Suffering from Water: Social Origins of Bodily Distress in a Mexican Community. Medical Anthropology Quarterly 15:3.

Erhart, E.M.
1997   Infant Death in Propithecus diadema edwardsi at Vatoharanana, RNPP, Madagascar. American Journal of Physical Anthropology, Supplement 24 (Annual Meeting Issue): 108.

Eriksen, Thomas Hylland
1993   Ethnicity and Nationalism: Anthropological Perspectives. London and Boulder: Pluto Press.

Erlich, Anne H. and Paul R. Erlich
1990   Life in Peril. In Lessons of the Rainforest. Edited y Suzanne Head
        and Robert Heinzman. San Francisco: Sierra Club Books.

Fairhead, James and Melissa Leach
1996   Rethinking the Forest-Savanna Mosaic: Colonial Science and its
        Relics in West Africa. In The Lie of the Land: Challenging Re-
        ceived Wisdom on the African Environment. Melissa Leach and
        Robin Mearns, Eds., pp. 105-121. Portsmouth, NH and Oxford:
        Heinemann.

Farmer, Paul
1999   Infections and Inequalities: The Modern Plagues, Updated Edi-
        tion. Berkeley: University of California Press.

1995   Aids and Accusation: Haiti and the Geography of Blame. Berke-
        ley and Los Angeles: University of California Press.

Feeley-Harnik, Gillian
1991   A Green Estate: Restoring Independence in Madagascar. Wash-
        ington and London: Smithsonian Institution Press.

1995   Plants and People, Children or Wealth: Shifting Grounds of
        "Choice" in Madagascar. PoLAR 18:2:45-64.

Feierman, Steven
1985   Struggles for Control: The Social Roots of Health and Healing in
        Modern Africa. African Studies Review 28:2/3:73-147.

Ferguson, James
1994   The Anti-Politics Machine. Minneapolis: University of Minnesota
        Press.

Ferraro, Paul John
1994   Natural Resource Use in the Southeastern Rain Forests of Mada-
        gascar and the Local Impacts of Establishing the Ranomafana Na-
        tional Park. M.S. Thesis, Department of the Environment, Duke
        University.

Ferraro, Paul and Basile Rakotondrajaona
1992   Preliminary Assessment of Local Population Forest Use, Forestry
        Initiatives, Agricultural Operations, Cultural Diversity, and the
        Potential for Rural Development in the Region of the Ranomafana
        National park, 1990-1991. In Socio-Economic Surveys in the Ra-
        nomafana National Park Periphery. Ranomafana National Park
        Project. Pp. 78-129. Durham: Duke University.

Foucault, Michel
1979   Discipline and Punish. Harmondsworth.

Frank, Andre Gundar
1969   Capitalism and Underdevelopment in Latin America: Historical Studies of Chili and Brazil. New York: Monthly Review Press.

Fraser, George MacDonald
1977   Flashman's Lady. New York: Alfred A. Knopf.

Gare, Arran E.
1995   Postmodernism and the Environmental Crisis. New York: Routledge.

Gershman, John and Alec Irwin
2000   Getting a Grip on the Global Economy. In Dying for Growth: Global Inequality and the Health of the Poor, Kim, Jim Yong, Joyce V. Millen, Alec Irwin, and John Gershman, Editors. pp. 11-43. Monroe, Maine: Common Courage Press.

Glick, Leonard B.
1967   Medicine as an Ethnographic Category: The Gimi of the New Guinea Highlands. Ethnology 6:31-56.

Gruenbaum, Ellen
1996   The Cultural Debate over Female Circumcision: The Sudanese Are Arguing This One Out for Themselves. Medical Anthropology Quarterly 10:4:455-475.

Hancock, Graham
1989   Lords of Poverty: The Power, Prestige, and Corruption of the International Aid Business. New York: The Atlantic Monthly Press.

Hanson, Paul
1993   Reconceiving the Shape of Culture: Folklore and Public Culture. Western Folklore 52:327-34

1997   The Politics of Need Interpretation in Madagascar's Ranomafana National Park. Ph.D. Dissertation, Department of Folklore and Folklife, University of Pennsylvania.

Hardenbergh, Sabrina
1992   Household Food Distribution of Subsistence Slash-and-Burn Cultivators near Ranomafana National Park, Madagascar. Presented at the Annual Meetings of the American Anthropological Association, San Francisco.

Harris, Marvin
1968 The Rise of Anthropological Theory: A History of Theories of Culture. New York: Thomas Crowell Company.

1979 Cultural Materialism: The Struggle for a Science of Culture. New York: Random House.

1992 Anthropology and the Theoretical and Paradigmatic Significance of the Collapse of Soviet and East European Communism. American Anthropologist 94:295-305.

1999 Theories of Culture in Postmodern Times. Walnut Creek: Alta Mira Press.

Harrison, Paul
1992 The Third Revolution: Population, Environment and a Sustainable World. London: Penguin Books.

Hecht, Susanna and Alexander Cockburn
1990 The Fate of the Forest: Developers, Destroyers and Defenders of the Amazon. New York: HarperPerennial.

Hemingway, C. A.
1996 Effects of Food Availability and Forest Composition on Feeding Patterns of Propithecus diadema edwardsi. American Journal of Physical Anthropology, Supplement 24 (Annual Meeting Issue):126.

Hildyard, Nicholas
1993 Foxes in Charge of the Chickens. In Global Ecology: A New Arena of Political Conflict. Wolfgang Sachs, Editor. London and New Jersey: Zed Books.

Howard, Mary Theresa and Ann Millard
1997 Hunger and Shame: Child Malnutrition and Poverty on Mt. Kilimanjaro. London and New York: Routledge.

Huntington, Richard
1988 Gender and Social Structure in Madagascar. Bloomington and Indianapolis: Indiana University Press.

Jarosz, Lucy Antonina
1993 Defining and Explaining Tropical Deforestation: Shifting Cultivation and Population Growth in Colonial Madagascar (1896-1940). Economic Geography 69:4:366-379.

Jolly, Alison
1987   Man Against Nature: Time for a Truce in Madagascar. National
        Geographic, February 1987:160-183.

Jordan, Brigitte
1993   Birth in Four Cultures: A Crosscultural Investigation of Child-
        birth in Yucatan, Holland, Sweden, and the United States, Fourth
        Edition. Prospect Heights: Waveland Press.

Keck, Andrew, Narendra P. Sharma and Gershon Feder
1994   Population Growth, Shifting Cultivation, and Unsustainable Agri-
        cultural Development: A Case Study in Madagascar. World Bank
        Discussion Papers #234. Africa Technical Department Series.

Kent, Raymond
1970   Early Kingdoms in Madagascar. New York: Holt, Rinehart.

Kightlinger, Lon K.
1993   Mechanisms of *Ascaris lumbricoides* Overdispersion in Human
        Communities in the Malagasy Rainforest. Ph.D. Dissertation. Uni-
        versity of North Carolina at Chapel Hill, North Carolina.

Kightlinger, L., M.B. Kightlinger, M. Rakotoaraivelo, J. Rakotonirina, S.
Ramarolahy, and V. Ravaohantaharinoro
1992   Socioeconomic and Health Aspects of Eighteen Communities Sur-
        rounding Ranomafana National Park, Madagascar, 1990-1991.
        In Socio-Economic Surveys in the Ranomafana National Park Pe-
        riphery. Ranomafana National Park Project.

Kim, Jim Yong, Joyce V. Millen, Alec Irwin, and John Gershman, Editors
2000   Dying for Growth: Global Inequality and the Health of the Poor.
        Monroe, Maine: Common Courage Press.

Knox, Margaret L.
1989   No Nation an Island. Sierra, May/June 1989:78-84.

Kottak, Conrad
1971a   Cultural Adaptation, Kinship, and Descent in Madagascar. South-
        western Journal of Anthropology 27:2:129-147.

1971b   Social Groups and Kinship Calculation Among the Southern Bet-
        sileo. American Anthropologists 73:178-193.

1980   The Past in the Present. Ann Arbor: The University of Michigan
        Press.

Larson, Pier Martin
1992   Making Ethnic Tradition in a Pre-Colonial Society: Culture, Gen-

der, and Protest in the Early Merina Kingdom, 1750-1822. Ph.D. Dissertation, University of Wisconsin-Madison.

1996   Desperately Seeking the 'Merina' (Central Madagascar): Reading Ethnonyms and Their Semantic Fields in African Identity Histories," Journal of Southern African Studies 22:4:541-560.

2000   History and Memory in the Age of Enslavement: Becoming Merina in Highland Madagascar, 1770-1882. Portsmouth, N. H.: Heinemann Social History of Africa Series.

Leacock, Eleanor Burke
1982   Marxism and Anthropology. In The Left Academy: Marxist Scholarship on American Campuses. B. Ollman and E. Vernoff, Eds. Pp. 242-276. New York: McGraw Hill.

Leatherman, Thomas
1996   A Biocultural Perspective on Health and Household Economy in Southern Peru. Medical Anthropology Quarterly 10:4:476-495.

Leisz, Stephen, Andrea Robles, and James Gage
1994   Land and Natural Resource Tenure and Security in Madagascar. Report prepared for USAID/Madagascar. Land Tenure Center, University of Wisconsin-Madison.

Linton, Ralph
1933   The Tanala: A Hill Tribe of Madagascar. Chicago: Field Museum of Natural History.

1939   Analysis of Tanala Culture. In The Individual and His Society. By Abram Kardiner, with a foreword and two ethnological reports by Ralph Linton. Pp. 291-354. New York: Columbia University Press.

1957   The Tree of Culture. New York: Alfred A. Knopf.

Lord, T.
1900   The Early History of Imerina Based Upon a Native Account. Antananarivo Annual VI:451475.

Mannoni, O.
1990   Prospero and Caliban: The Psychology of Colonization. Ann Arbor: The University of Michigan Press.

Mayer, Jonathan D.
1996   The Political Ecology of Disease as One New Focus for Medical Geography. Progress in Human Geography 20:4:441-456.

2000   Geography, Ecology, and Emerging Infectious Diseases. Social Science and Medicine 50:7-8:937-952.

McCaleb, Robert S.
1997   Medicinal Plants for Healing the Planet: Biodiversity and Environmental Health Care. In Biodiversity and Human Health, Francesca Grifo and Joshua Rosenthal, Eds. Pp. 221-242. Washington, D.C.: Island Press.

McCay, Bonnie J. and James M. Acheson, Eds.
1987   The Question of the Commons: The Culture and Ecology of Communal Resources. Tucson: University of Arizona Press.

McElroy, Ann and Patricia K. Townsend
1996   Medical Anthropology in Ecological Perspective, Third Edition. Boulder: Westview Press.

McNeely, Jeffrey A. and Sara J. Scherr
2001   Common Ground, Common Future: How Ecoagriculture can Help Feed the World and Save Wild Biodiversity. Washington, D.C. and Gland, Switzerland: The World Conservation Union (IUCN) and Future Harvest Report [available online at http://www.future-harvest.org/pdf/biodiversity_report.pdf]

Middleton, Neil, Phil O'Keefe and Sam Moyo
1993   Tears of the Crocodile: From Rio to Reality in the Developing World. London and Boulder: Pluto Press.

Millard, Ann V.
1992   The Anthropological Analysis of Health. Medical Anthropology Quarterly 6:1:3-5.

Millen, Joyce V., Alec Irwin, and Jim Yong Kim
2000   Introduction: What is Growing? Who is Dying? In Dying for Growth: Global Inequality and the Health of the Poor, Kim, Jim Yong, Joyce V. Millen, Alec Irwin, and John Gershman, Editors. pp. 3-10. Monroe, Maine: Common Courage Press.

Milton, Kay
1996   Environmentalism and Culture Theory: Exploring the Role of Anthropology in Environmental Discourse. London and New York: Routledge.

Morgan, Lynn M.
1984   Dependency Theory in the Political Economy of Health An Anthropological Critique. Medical Anthropology Quarterly 1(2):131-153.

Morsy, Soheir
1979   The Missing Link in Medical Anthropology: The Political Economy of Health. Reviews in Anthropology 6:349-363.

1996   Political Economy in Medical Anthropology. In Medical Anthropology: Contemporary Theory and Method, Revised Edition. Edited by Carolyn F. Sargent and Thomas M. Johnson. pp.21-40. Westport and London: Praeger.

Murphy, Dervla
1985   Muddling Through in Madagascar. Woodstock: The Overlook Press.

Naranjo, Plutarco
1995   Archaeology and Psychoactive Plants. In Ethnobotany: Evolution of a Discipline. Richard Evans Schultes and Siri von Reis, Eds., pp.393-399. Portland, Oregon: Dioscorides Press.

Oxby, Clare
1985   Forest Farmers: The Transformation of Land Use and Society in Eastern Madagascar. Unasylva 37:2:42-51.

Peters, Dai
1994a   Indigenous Healing and its Role in Health Care in the Ranomafana National Park Periphery of Madagascar. Paper presented at the Symposium on Indigenous Knowledge and Contemporary Social Issues. Tampa: University of Southern Florida, March 14-16, 1994.

1994b   Social Impact Assessment of the Ranomafana National Park Project of Madagascar. Paper presented at the International Association of Impact Assessment conference in Quebec City, Canada, 14-17 June 1994.

Peters, William Joseph, Jr.
1997   Local Participation in Conservation of the Ranomafana National Park, Madagascar. Journal of World Forest Resource Management 8:109-135.

1999   Transforming the Integrated Conservation and Development Project (ICDP) Approach: Observations from the Ranomafana National Park Project, Madagascar. Agriculture and Human Values 16:1:65-74.

Plotkin, Mark
1993   Tales of a Shaman's Apprentice: An Ethnobotanist Searches for New Medicines in the Amazon Rain Forest. New York: Viking.

Pryor, Frederic L.
1990   The Political Economy of Poverty, Equity, and Growth: Malawi and Madagascar. Washington: Oxford University Press (for the World Bank).

Quammen, David
1991   A Murder in Madagascar. Audubon 93:1:48-58.

Rabetaliana, Hanta
n/d   Prospects for Natural Resource Management in Madagascar. Unpublished Manuscript, WorldWide Fund for Nature, Antananarivo, Madagascar.

Ranomafana National Park
1994   Ranomafana National Park: Integrated Conservation and Development Project 1994-1996. Stoney Brook: Ranomafana National Park Project.

Rhodes, Lorna Amarasingham
1996   Studying Biomedicine as a Medical System. In Medical Anthropology: Contemporary Theory and Method, Revised Edition. Edited by Carolyn F. Sargent and Thomas M. Johnson. pp. 165-182. Westport and London: Praeger.

Sampan' Asa Fambolena Fiombiana (SAFAFI)
1989   Survey of Ranomafana Park Pilot Villages. Unpublished document submitted to Dr. Patricia Wright, Ranomafana National Park Conservation Project, September 26, 1989.

Schmink, Marianne and Charles H. Wood
1987   The "Political Ecology" of Amazonia. In Lands at Risk in the Third World: Local-Level Perspectives, Edited by Peter D. Little, Michael M. Horowitz and A. Endre Nyerges, pp. 38-57. Boulder: Westview Press.

Sharp, Lesley A.
1993   The Possessed and the Dispossessed: Spirits, Identity, and Power in a Madagascar Migrant Town. Berkeley: University of California Press.

Shiva, Vandana
1991   The Violence of the Green Revolution: Third World Agriculture, Ecology and Politics. London and New Jersey: Zed Books, Ltd.

Sibree, James
1878   The Sakalava: Their Origin, Conquests, and Subjugation; A Chapter in Malagasy History. Antananarivo Annual I:456-468.

Singer, Merrill
1986   Toward a Political-Economy of Alcoholism: The Missing Link in the Anthropology of Drinking. Social Science & Medicine 23(2):113-130.

Stevens, Rita
1999   Madagascar. Philadelphia: Chelsea House Publishers.

Steward, Julien
1955   Theory of Culture Change: The Methodology of Multilinear Evolution. Urbana: University of Illinois Press.

Stewart, Pamela J. and Andrew Strathern
2000   Discussions on Consultancy and Anthropology. Okari Research Group Prepublication Working Paper, No. 17.

Stoner, Bradley P.
1986   Understanding Medical Systems: Traditional, Modern, and Syncretic Health Care Alternatives in Medically Pluralistic Societies. Medical Anthropology Quarterly 17:2:44-48.

Strathern, Andrew and Pamela J. Stewart
1999   Curing and Healing: Medical Anthropology in Global Perspective. Durham: Carolina Academic Press.

Sustainable Approaches to Viable Environmental Management (SAVEM)
1997   Madagascar's Integrated Conservation and Development Projects: Lessons Learned by Participants, Project Employees, Related Authorities and Community Beneficiaries. Executive Summary, May, 1997. Submitted by K. Lynn McCoy and Hajanirina Razafindrainibe.

Sussman, Linda K.
1988   Routine Herbal Treatment for Pregnant Women, Neonates, and Postpartum Care Among the Mahafaly of Southwest Madagascar. Unpublished manuscript of presentation at the Annual Meeting of the American Anthropological Association, Phoenix, Arizona, November 1988.

Systematics Agenda 2000: Charting the Biosphere
1993   New York: American Museum of Natural History.

Tacchi, A.
1892   King Andrianampoinimerina, and the Early History of Antananarivo and Ambohimanga. Antananarivo Annual IV:474-496.

Taussig, Michael
1980   Reification and the Consciousness of the Patient. Social Science and Medicine 14B:3-13.

Thébault, E. P.
1951   *Traité de Droit Civil Malgache: Les Lois et Coutumes Hova. Fascicule II: Les Biens, Les Obligations et Les Contrats.* Paris: Jouve & Co., *E'diteurs.*

UNICEF.
1992.   State of the World's Children. Oxford, UK: Oxford University Press.

United States Agency for International Development (USAID)
n/d   USAID/Madagascar Environment Program. USAID, Antanarivo.

2001   Madagascar. http://www.usaid.gov/country/afr/mg/ dated: January 23, 2001

van der Geest, Sjaak, and Susan R. Whyte, Editors
1988   The Context of Medicines in Developing Countries. Dordrecht: Kluwer Academic Publishers.

Vandermeer, John and Ivette Perfecto
1995   Breakfast of Biodiversity: The Truth About Rain Forest Destruction. Oakland: Institute for Food and Development Policy.

Vaughan, Megan
1991   Curing Their Ills: Colonial Power and African Illness. Stanford: Stanford University Press.

Vayda, Andrew P. and Bradley B. Walters
1999   Against Political Ecology. Human Ecology 27:1:167-179.

Vérin, Pierre
1990   Madagascar. Paris: Karthala Press.

1986   The History of Civilisation in North Madagascar. Translated by David Smith. Rotterdam and Boston: A. A. Balkema.

Warren, Michael
1997   Employment and Income-Generating for Indigenous and Tribal Peoples: Lessons Learned in Asia. Unpublished manuscript presented at ILO-INDISCO Donor Consultation and Planning Workshop. New Delhi, India, 4-8 November 1997.

Watts, Michael
1989   The Agrarian Question in Africa: Debating the Crisis. Progress in Human Geography 17:257-272.

World Bank
1994   Madagascar: A Strategy for High Growth and Poverty Alleviation: An Economic Strategy Note. Report No. 13274-MAG, June

29, 1994, Country Operations Division, South Asia and Indian Ocean Department, Africa Region.

1996   Office Memorandum, for General Distribution, from Nils O. Tcheyan, Chief, AF3AE, Dated February 23, 1996, Re: Madagascar—Proposed Second Environment Program Support Project, Pre-appraisal Review Meeting.

World Health Organization
1988   Ethical Criteria for Medicinal Drug Promotion. Geneva: World Health Organization.

Wright, Patricia C.
1990   Ecosystem Preservation and Public Health. Environmental Impact Assessment Review 10:451-453.

1992   Primate Ecology, Rainforest Conservation, and Economic Development: Building a National Park in Madagascar. Evolutionary Anthropology 1:1:25-33.

1993   Ranomafana National Park, Madagascar: Rainforest Conservation and Economic Development. Prepared for the Liz Claiborne-Art Ortenberg Foundation Community-Based Conservation Workshop, Arlie, Virginia, 18-22 October 1993.

Wright, P.C., D.M. Haring, M.K. Izard, and E.L. Simons.
1989   Psychological Well-Being of Nocturnal Primates in Captivity. In E. F. Segal (Ed.), Housing, Care and Psychological Wellbeing of Captive and Laboratory Primates (pp. 61-74). Parkridge: Noyes Publications.

Young, Crawford
1986   Nationalism, Ethnicity, and Class in Africa. *Cahiers d'Etudes Africaines* 26:3:453.

Zerner, Charles
1996   "Telling Stories about Biological Diversity," pp. 68-101 in Valuing Local Knowledge: Indigenous People and Intellectual Property Rights, Stephen B. Brush and Doreen Stabinsky, Eds. Washington, D.C.: Island Press.

Index